No Time For Cancer

NO TIME FOR CANCER

Inspire Yourself to Survive Mouth, Head and Neck Cancer

Carol Dunstone & Ann Bennett

Matador
9 Priory Business Park
Kibworth Beauchamp
Leicestershire LE8 0RX, UK
Tel: (+44) 116 279 2299
Fax: (+44) 116 279 2277
Email: books@troubador.co.uk
Web: www.troubador.co.uk/matador

ISBN 978-1783061-228

British Library Cataloguing in Publication Data.
A catalogue record for this book is available from the British Library.

Typeset in Aldine by Troubador Publishing Ltd
Printed and bound in the UK by TJ International, Padstow, Cornwall

Matador is an imprint of Troubador Publishing Ltd

For Ann

ACKNOWLEDGMENTS

Carol and Ann would like to thank everyone who helped them throughout their journeys from diagnosis to recovery and their continuing journey. They especially thank their families for their constant support.

Carol's husband, children and sisters. Ann's husband, children and sister.

They also thank their dear friends for their support throughout, those who contributed recipes and all those named specialists who contributed articles. And they give special thanks to their consultants and medical teams.

They would also like to thank all those (many people) involved with setting up and supporting the Dunstone Bennett Complementary Centre (DB) – the management teams, therapists and receptionists, including all the Trustees for our charity Facefax: Anne Hicks, Gordon and Sophie Chandler, Pauline Gibbings, Jean Patchesa, Joyce Turner and Bill Dearns

Finally they would like to thank all those involved in helping to produce this book – Tony Boullemier, Inga Sutton, Brian Dunstone (Bunny), Elsa Christie, Michael Bennett, Vicky Smith, Sue Brooks and Christine Owens. Elke Pollard and Roger Wilkin.

They would also like to express special thanks to Macmillan, the Freemasons of Northamptonshire, Huntingdonshire and Buckinghamshire, Nigella Lawson and Professor Nick Stafford for their interest and support.

CONTENTS

INTRODUCTION

THE AUTHORS

Carol Dunstone is a ceramic artist and had a full-time career, designing, painting and producing ceramics, until cancer of the mouth was diagnosed in 1998.

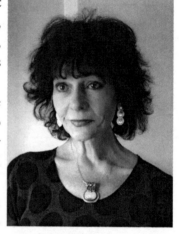

She lives in Northamptonshire with her husband Brian, known to everyone as Bunny. She is the mother of three children, Alastair, Clare and James, and has seven grandchildren.

Her ceramic art continues and she works at home in her own studio along with Bunny who is a sculptor. Her interests include painting, reading, gardening, walking the dog and family life.

Carol was making a good recovery from her illness when, in 2001, she helped set up Facefax, a support group for head and neck cancer patients. There she met Ann Bennett and together they discussed how they could use their own experiences to collate information and provide tips and suitable cooking recipes for fellow patients and their families.

Three years ago, Carol and Ann set up a therapy centre for all cancer patients and supporters. Carol now teaches art at the DB.

Ann Bennett, born in Wiltshire, now lives in Northampton. She is married to Michael and has a thirty-eight-year-old-son, Mark. She also has an extended family, Vicky Golding and husband Oscar, their two children and Vicky's brother, Max and partner Rumi. Ann's interests include entertainment, travel and reading.

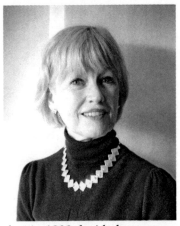

For many years Ann worked in the business world and in advertising, but in 1993 decided to pursue her interest in complementary therapies and trained as an Advanced Reiki practitioner. She became a full member with the National Federation of Spiritual Healers and qualified as an Advanced Hypnotherapist and Hypno-Healer. She has incorporated all three therapies within the book and for the Dunstone Bennett Complementary Centre. Ann was fifty-six when diagnosed with mouth cancer in 2004. Eight months after her operation she met Carol when she attended her first Facefax meeting.

After much encouragement, both Carol and Ann have updated their journeys, continuing from 2006 until now, with many new contributions. Much progress has been made in the passing years, which they hope will highlight a very definite and positive outlook for their readers with this new book.

FOREWORD

PROFESSOR STAFFORD

To be diagnosed with cancer is a devastating event in anyone's life. As a Head and Neck Surgeon, I have always got the impression that patients regard tumours of the upper airway and digestive tract as the most difficult to deal with. Not only do they have a cancer, but they have something which is very close to their very being and which is likely to cause cosmetic, swallowing or voice disruption. Unfortunately, none of these can be easily disguised from friends and relatives in the same way a breast or colon cancer can.

There are many books written about head and neck cancer, but most of them are written by members of the medical profession and deal objectively with how the physician should manage the tumour. However, it is really only the patient who knows the best way to cope with the diagnosis and how best to live with it. Carol and Ann have written about such issues in a way that will be very helpful to others undergoing the treatment and problems that they experienced themselves. Knowledge is no substitute for experience and this book provides a summary of all the thoughts and events a person with oral cavity cancer is going to go through during their treatment. It can be thought of as a frontline battle tale as opposed to a manual of military strategy.

I would whole-heartedly recommend this book to anyone with an interest, either personal or general, in this area of oncology.

Chapter 1

HOW FACEFAX STARTED

"Being told you have cancer or that your cancer has returned or can't be cured, can leave you feeling shocked, upset and very isolated. There are so many feelings to deal with and it can be a very confusing and distressing time."
The Macmillan Cancer Line

The Facefax support group was first established in Northampton in June 2001 when it became apparent that many patients with mouth, head and neck cancer were not getting enough support on their journeys towards recovery.

When Carol Dunstone mentioned to her consultant Mr Clive Pratt that there seemed to be a lack of immediate contact and backup for patients like herself, he agreed. He suggested she meet another patient named Valerie Johal who was recovering from mouth cancer. When she and Carol met, they found their experiences gave them a close bond.

They began meeting other patients about once a month at Northampton General Hospital, with Sister Jane Bradley acting as facilitator. Their aim was to provide information and support to patients and carers, and as the group grew, it was registered as a charity, The Facefax Association.

The association's main aim is to increase public and professional awareness of these cancers.

Anne Hicks now acts as the Facefax facilitator. She gives up much of her time listening to patients' problems and is always full of advice. The group regards her as indispensable.

A Unique Link

By Anne Hicks, Maxillofacial Clinical Nurse Specialist, Northampton General Hospital

My patients are all undergoing treatment for head and neck cancer and since the diagnosis usually comes out of the blue, it is liable to leave them in a complete state of shock. But I will be present at the point of diagnosis and will be their point of contact in the hospital throughout their treatment.

I ensure that my patients and their loved ones get information about their planned treatment and offer emotional support as required. I encourage them to ask questions and discuss the life-changing experience they are having.

Verbal information is supported by a written information pack and given over two or three forty-five minute consultations. It is important that patients and their loved ones understand all the treatment options and give their informed consent. Every patient will require different levels of information given at their own pace. As doctors and nurses, we know that too much information given too soon after a diagnosis of cancer will not be understood, leading to problems later in the recovery process.

I manage all wounds following surgery and take part in the review process in conjunction with my medical colleagues. Consequently, the relationship with my patients will hopefully last at least five years.

I am chairman of Facefax and also facilitate the Facefax support group meetings held in Northampton. Only a small percentage of my patients attend regularly, but those who do are so full of energy and enthusiasm.

Chapter 2

CAROL'S STORY: MY DIARY

INTRODUCTION

No time for cancer. Where have all those years gone? I was diagnosed with mouth cancer fifteen years ago, when I underwent twelve hours of surgery, followed by six weeks of radiation treatment and here I am now beginning another journey.

I am writing a second book with my dear friend and co-author, Ann Bennett. By popular request, this book is to follow where we left off six years ago after the publication of our first book called *TRILOGY*.

We can't influence the past, so maybe we can influence the future. We must continue to go forward and learn. As one gets older, the essence of friendship is ever more intense with the knowledge of either moving on.

I'm tracing my footsteps back to 2005, reawakening memories, both happy and joyful, but also sad. This has been quite cathartic for me.

In 2005, I already had three grandchildren, Connor, Clare's son, and Libiana and William, Alastair and Vanessa's children. Later that same year, Sophie, my fourth grandchild, was born in Canada to James, my youngest son, and his wife, Melissa. In the Autumn, I flew out to Calgary with my daughter, Clare, and grandson, Connor, to visit my latest grandchild. This was such an exciting trip and it was a beautiful time of year, with all the changing colours of the

Fall, bursts of warm sunshine and then, in such contrast, heavy snow. That was my first trip to Calgary; but not the first to Canada.

We had all gone out to celebrate James and Lis's marriage in Saskatoon the summer before. On the night of the open-air wedding party, the Canadian sky turned into brilliant colours, moving and shifting around. This was the Aurora Borealis or the Merry Dancers as they are called in Orkney – a truly magical vision and, to all those who witnessed it, a very special omen.

To round off our stay in Saskatoon, the wedding party, including all the families on both sides, made a long trek to a huge national park, far north in Canada. We stayed in individual wooden chalets dotted about in a densely wooded area near the Lake of the Loons, in the middle of nowhere. My body rushed with adrenalin as I read signs; signs warning of bears, cougars, wolves and coyotes all indigenous to the area. This was the most incredible place, far away from human habitation and so very wild. In fact, the road beyond us literally ran out into a vast area of wilderness, stretching on eventually to the Arctic. Much to my delight, I found a place called Orkney on the map; but we didn't get there.

I'll never forget the intense deep blackness as the night closed in; the hundreds of stars so near; the primal sounds of wolves howling in the distance so close to touching our basic being – so wild and such an awareness of our solitude. How small man is. This I knew was part of the healing process after the nightmarish traumas I had been through. I have to add on a lighter note – the only wild animal I saw was a porcupine!

I've had many trips over to Canada since and always feel such a thrill upon arrival. If only I could do it more often; but we do all try to meet up as a family in the UK as often as we can. The joys of our children living overseas!

Travelling for me is quite nerve-wracking. I always worry about not having enough water, because I get such a dry mouth. I literally dry up – become tongue-tied – enabling my speech to become quite a problem. I worry if I will be able to eat the food on the plane, despite notifying the airline in advance, and invariably the answer is no. I can manage some soft foods, like a yoghurt or ice cream, but it is not easy. Of course, on a short flight it is much easier to cope with. Unfortunately the FORTISIPS, which are my fail safe supplementary nutritional drinks cannot be carried on board (these may be obtained on prescription). There must be a way around this – perhaps I haven't persevered enough. Anyway, I know I won't starve. I used to panic about not being able to eat when out in public; but now I either eat in advance at home, because it takes so long to swallow a meal, or I eat when I get back home. At least it saves a lot of embarrassment for all and I can relax and enjoy myself. These problems with dry mouth and swallowing are a legacy of radical surgery and radiation treatment.

Dry mouth must be one of the main problems following surgery on the mouth, head and neck. Night time can be difficult. I use a gel called BIOTENE for relief of dry mouth, plenty of water by the bedside and now a new tip provided by the Maxillofacial Clinic – olive oil can be rubbed very lightly around the inside of the mouth and on the lips. Doesn't taste too good and a bit messy – but effective. Not exactly the most flattering look for my long-suffering husband! I'm also very aware of dental hygiene – which is so important. On recommendation, I use special toothpaste at night called DURAPHAT 5000 ppm with fluoride and a special dental tooth mousse. Please do ask your dentist first before using this.

Another hazard when going through customs is that I always set off the alarm button. Inevitably a body search is followed, which makes me feel quite indignant at times – however, I am much resigned to the search now. I do try to explain I still have a plate screwed into my lower jawbone. This essential procedure took place when I had my tumour removed from the tonsil area and back of the throat. My face had to be divided in two, to allow access for the surgery which took place. As a result, my jawbone was broken and later held in place with small plates and screws. One plate was removed not long after the main operation, as it had shifted, but the other is still in place. One would never know, such is the marvel of modern surgery and the dedicated medical teams and surgeons who worked to save my life. I'm incredibly grateful to them all, especially Mr Pratt and Mr Smith, my two maxillofacial surgeons.

The only clue to those aware of the massive amount of surgery I had is perhaps my slight speech impediment. I do find I often have to explain, especially if talking on the telephone to people who don't know me. This can lead to many scrapes, so I often just say I've just come back from the dentist – a little white lie? However, it does help.

Some years ago I attended a party in the village, where I had what my friends now call a 'Red Glub' moment! At the end of the party, I spent an anxious time trying to find my new red leather gloves. They seemed to have vanished into thin air. I know I am absent-minded but this disappearance turned into a major search, and the more I tried to explain, the harder the word 'gloves' became. Tony, our friend and editor of our first book, thought this was hilarious – hence 'Red Glubs' has been fondly adopted and now has a special meaning for my difficult moments!

Early in the summer of 2005, my husband Bunny and I travelled north to Orkney and it was during this particular visit that we made a momentous decision. The decision to actually move our lives away from the midlands in the heart of England and settle in a wonderful old house with land and space all around. This house in Orkney was nestled on a hillside with wide open skies and seas, and was so totally different from our cottage in Boughton.

Later that holiday on our way south, we met up with family and friends at a very large Scottish house near Inverness called Invereshie. We had a lovely week with everyone there, excitedly discussing our new plans.

Returning home, however, and as time went on, the thought of selling up – we had put our house on the market – leaving family and friends, began to outweigh heavily on our decision. By this time Bunny had stopped working, retiring early from his full-time career as Director of Design for a large furniture company. We were in limbo and I know the uncertainty of our future wreaked havoc on our health. Finally, the decision was made for us – the vendors backed out of the sale and it was only then that the feeling of regret, but also relief, came into play. After all, we still had 'The Noust', our small cottage situated in Stromness, as somewhere to stay whenever we visited Orkney.

But what now? Both being artists we knew we would struggle to make a living, but somehow we have and still enjoy our lives immensely.

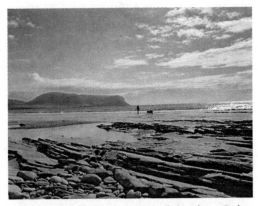

Walking with the dogs at Warbeth beach in Orkney

A CHAPTER OF EVENTS

First I must explain what happened to me in 1998, when it was confirmed I had mouth cancer. I had previously been fully occupied working as a ceramic artist, designing, teaching and painting for a well-established British ceramic company, working with and designing for many major stores such as Harrods, Selfridges, Liberty, Conran and John Lewis. We also designed ceramics for the Fauve Exhibition at the Royal Academy and for the National Gallery in London. We worked with such famous people as Marco Pierre White, Gordon Ramsay and Cameron Mackintosh. I flew to Japan to demonstrate ceramic painting and we exhibited our designs at major stores in Tokyo. All of which was very stimulating and exciting. I had a very busy life with three teenage children at home and working full time.

However, on my return from Tokyo I began to feel quite unwell. I had developed earache, a sore jaw and an ulcerated mouth – all of which was dragging me down and making me feel extremely tired. I made an appointment to see my GP and was very surprised when it was recommended I should have a second opinion. This was duly arranged and within a short period of time I had an appointment to see Mr Clive Pratt, the Maxillofacial consultant based at Woodlands Hospital in Kettering.

I was relieved that something at last was happening and after an examination and an x-ray of the jaw and neck area, Mr Pratt said he would like to admit me for a minor operation. At this stage, I had no idea anything too serious was amiss and no one had mentioned the word 'cancer'.

The results of my so-called 'minor op' were back in days – apparently it had turned out to be a three-hour operation in the end!

Bunny, my partner then, now my husband, came with me to

see Mr Pratt for the results. It was devastating news. Everyone there was very kind, but I only remember feeling so isolated trying to digest the terrible news. Poor Bunny looked shattered. We hardly dared to look at each other. The atmosphere in the room was charged with concern.

I was diagnosed with a grade three tumour, which was situated in the tonsil area at the back of my throat. It was malignant, but it was hoped it was the primary tumour. Mr Pratt explained very carefully that this would mean a 'Belt and Braces' approach. Surgery to remove the tumour, followed by radiotherapy. This advice was to be very positive and Mr Pratt said he knew from experience that there were two choices, either turn my face to the wall (i.e. give up) or turn away from the wall and fight. How true those words are.

After endless check-ups, MRI scans and a feeding tube, (known as a 'PEG') inserted into my stomach, I was ready and prepared for my admittance to Kettering General Hospital – awaiting my 'big' operation.

The 'PEG' was an absolute necessity and literally proved a lifesaver in the months to come, especially during and after my radiation treatment.

Shockingly, I learned that I would have my lower jaw broken in two, to gain access to the tumour at the back of my tongue in the tonsil area. Then my lower face would be opened up, rather like the pages of a book. I would have lymph glands removed from my neck and I would lose one third of my tongue. I was to have a large flap of skin/tissue/muscle/veins (called a free flap) taken from my lower left arm (I'm right-handed) – and this would be removed by another surgeon, Mr Bill Smith. In other words, they would rebuild my throat with my arm. To replace the surgical wound on my arm, another skin graft was to be taken from my forearm.

Fortunately, I don't have very hairy arms; but much later I would meet other fellow patients who would joke with some hilarity about their tickly, hairy throats. I understand that this does not last forever, thank heavens.

There was still more to come as a large area of muscle would be affected in the shoulder area and I realised my left arm/shoulder and neck area would be out of action for a while. I did require considerable physiotherapy for several months, which happily improved the situation significantly. I will return to this later in my story.

I was also warned of the possibility of my jawbone being affected by more cancerous cells and if this was discovered, bone would be removed from my thigh bone and grafted into a 'new' jawbone. So apparently my body parts had many uses, welded into new places here and there. Skin grafts could also be a problem. Sometimes rejection might take place and a new area would have to be found, maybe high in the chest area or at the side of the temple area. Fortunately, my skin grafts and transplants worked and healed quite rapidly.

My teeth were another concern – perhaps I'm vain but Mr Pratt assured me he would try to save my teeth, and indeed he did a brilliant job.

When I had my operation, it did last twelve hours and it was two days before I was brought back gently into a state of consciousness. However, unfortunately I had a major setback resulting in a stay in Intensive Care for six days. The nursing staff were wonderful, so compassionate, patient and caring, and I can't thank them all enough. This dedicated team nursed me back to health. I must add that now, fifteen years later, much has moved on in the name of progress, enabling head, neck and mouth cancer patients to recover more rapidly.

Six weeks after my operation, I started my radiation treatment. This was five days a week for six weeks. Gruelling though it was, it was an essential part of my 'get well' treatment – the 'braces' part of treatment for my recovery. Looking back now, I realise it probably took a year to feel more like myself again and at least two years before I could happily feel it was a new beginning. During that year after all my surgery, I am so happy to say Bunny and I married in Orkney in my late mother's house on her birthday. A very special occasion for us and all the family. What a gift life is. More detail of my story is related in the first book *TRILOGY*, the pre-cursor to *NO TIME FOR CANCER*.

ON THE ROAD TO RECOVERY

Well on the road to recovery after my surgery, I tried to find other patients who had (also) experienced the same surgery I had. I met Valerie Johal, who was a patient of Mr Clive Pratt, and we discussed the possibility of setting up a support group. This gradually began to take shape, encouraging other mouth/head and neck cancer patients to come along and have a chat, some refreshment and perhaps listen to an invited speaker. And so began the birth of Facefax, which is now our registered charity for all mouth/head and neck cancer patients in Northamptonshire.

This was eventually how and where I met Annie. We instantly hit it off – recognising a kindred spirit in each other, resulting in a special and deep friendship. At last we found we could have a laugh and enjoy many situations which hitherto might have proved somewhat daunting – especially considering the many problems involved with the outcome of such invasive surgery. No explanations needed really if either one of us had a coughing fit or choked over our coffee and cake. Indeed, Ann and I still meet regularly on a monthly basis. We always sit in the coffee lounge at `Dreams` in St. Giles Street, where we are warmly welcomed by the proprietor, Mike Smith. We enjoy shopping together, have meals together and when our two husbands met, a new friendship was formed between us all. This helped enormously with many a problem Ann or I might be concerned with, regarding our former illness. We gave each other confidence and a real boost, which ultimately led to earnest discussions on writing a book together to help other cancer patients.

During the early months of 2006, such excitement was experienced – we finally had a publisher and Ann and I started to write our very first book together. This book was called *TRILOGY*: *How to help the Mind, Body and Spirit survive Mouth, Head and Neck Cancer*. In the early Spring, Bunny and I and my sister Inga flew to Spain to stay with my cousin Heulyn, who lives near Periana. What better place to encourage me to write the first chapter in such a wonderful and peaceful environment.

A frantically busy year ensued and as the summer moved on, our book took shape and was at last ready to be printed. We gave grateful thanks to all those many friends and helpers – without whom it would ever have materialised.

With much trepidation, Annie and I went to see the printers on the very day they had actually printed the first copy. Upon our arrival, everyone came out to greet us and congratulate us – clapping and cheering. It was such an experience, moving us to tears of elation and happiness.

Thrilled with the publication, Ann and I had a major book launch on 30th October in Northampton – a date we now celebrate every year. Our book launch was hugely supported and I know we both found this a very humbling experience. At last we were raising massive public awareness concerning mouth, head and neck cancer, which is now very much on the increase and worryingly affecting much younger people as well.

October that year was certainly a busy month. We had the

book launch, book signings and the thrill of seeing our book on the bookshelves. Indeed on a special trip to the main branch of Waterstones in London, we could hardly contain our excitement on seeing *TRILOGY* sitting on their shelves. This resulted in a quick dash around the corner for a congratulatory glass of champagne.

After all the excitement of the 'The Book', Bunny and I travelled north to Dalnagairn in Perthshire where my sister Inga was celebrating her sixtieth birthday with many other members of our large family joining her. I couldn't possibly have imagined such happiness a few years before, whilst I was recovering from cancer. I was now feeling fit and well, albeit coping with everyday speech and swallowing issues – but they seemed relatively minor in the bigger scheme of life.

November arrived with another grandchild on the way. Isabella, Bella as she is known, was born that month – a very beautiful sister for Connor. Then James and Melissa arrived from Canada with Sophie to spend Christmas with us all. Lis was pregnant with Ben, who was born the next February and shared the same birthday date as Bunny's. Vanessa and Alastair proudly announced the expectation of their third child and Isobel was born a few days after Ben. Three new grandchildren – wow – what a joy! Looking back to when I was first diagnosed with mouth cancer, it had certainly crossed my mind I might not have been here to enjoy a future of any kind with my family. But here I was, alive and relishing every minute. 'Dancing the Dance' as they say!

Four years later, we had to make the very sad and difficult decision to sell our cottage in Orkney. This was hugely devastating, especially for me, as it had been a symbol of hope and recovery when we first bought it, just after I was recovering from my radiotherapy treatment. However, it had to be done as it was becoming increasingly impossible to care for – logistics winning the day. I do miss our small house so much; but the lovely compensation is that Judy and John – my baby sister and her husband – still have a place there called 'Little Bu' and this is where we now stay as often as is possible. It certainly helps to ease the heartache I felt at the time of the loss, as Judy is always the ever generous hostess embracing our visits as she also loves to be there as often as she can be. Little Bu is much cherished by the family and this is where I am now writing this chapter.

Before I move on, I must recall a very amusing incident which happened during the time we stayed in our house in Stromness. This long journey north, 650 miles by car, was always broken with a night or two with Inga and her family who then still lived in Edinburgh, before driving all the way up to Thurso to catch the evening ferry across the Pentland Firth to Orkney. The excitement I always felt then and now, on arrival, never goes away. Our house was situated right on the seafront overlooking Scapa Flow. The sounds of birds and sea and yes – the wind – all deeply embedded in me.

However, we arrived on this occasion tired and hungry before falling into a fitful sleep. We still had our rather elderly Jack Russell terrier called Amy with us and whilst having breakfast the next morning, I absent-mindedly popped what I mistakenly believed to be my pills into my mouth and swallowed them! Then, horror of horrors, I realised I had actually swallowed Amy's pills and panic ensued. My husband rushed out to find the chemist, which was only just opening up. "Quick, quick, my wife has swallowed our dog's pills!" This had the immediate effect of producing much mirth and amusement by all in the shop. "Woof Woof" they all chorused, and from then on I was known as "that barking mad woman". Ha, ha. Fortunately for me I didn't come to any harm, although I do believe my 'growl' has got stronger, and maybe my nose is a little shinier!

LAUGHTER IS THE BEST MEDICINE

Following the success of our book *TRILOGY*, Ann and I busied ourselves with the task of marketing, raising funds and giving talks whenever and wherever possible. We had many functions such as a local charity barn dance; a fashion show hosted by Voni Blu, Northampton; the Sun at Hardingstone kindly let us use their premises for two events. We had a garden lunch party at Dallington Manor and a wonderful 'Big Ball' was organised by friends in the village.

These funds were all being raised for the Facefax charity – but also for another idea and project forming in our minds. Anne Hicks, Ann Bennett and I had been discussing a new idea for some time – but how to set about it? We wanted to set up a complementary therapy centre for not only head, neck and mouth cancer patients, but for all cancer patients, their families and carers. This was a dream about to become a reality.

In the meantime Ann and I talked to many different groups within the country, including medical groups and other organisations such as libraries, local clubs – in fact, wherever we could get a foot in the door! This at times proved to be quite hilarious; endorsing the fact that laughter is really a very positive approach, albeit such a serious subject. We do make a good team together, 'Tweedle Dum and Tweedle Dee', and I know that it certainly helped us both to manage certain difficulties which can crop up. We try very hard to explain the problems and difficulties that we have both incurred with mouth cancer, but hopefully remain positive and upbeat as well.

The main thing is, we are making people aware of the importance of early detection and diagnosis of mouth, head and neck cancers. Early detection means survival and this cannot be emphasised enough. It is amazing how unaware and how little knowledge the general public have about this cancer. The British Dental Health Foundation, in a survey carried out in 2007, found that one in four people have never even heard of mouth cancer. Fifty years ago, mouth cancer was five times more common in men than women. Now, it is only twice as common.

Then, out of the blue, following all our talks and fundraising efforts, an amazing thing happened. Arthur Piggins, a very special friend of mine, who on behalf of the Freemasons had been liaising with Northampton General Hospital raising funds for them, asked to see me. He explained he might be able to help us find a room within the hospital, which might suit our purposes. He had become very interested in our idea of establishing a centre for cancer patients. A meeting was duly arranged at the Cripps Social Club at the Northampton General Hospital, where we were introduced to Keith Brooks in charge of financial control at NGH. He arrived with his secretary and Anne Hicks, our Chairman of Facefax, Arthur, Bunny and myself, including the manager of the Cripps Club, all sat down to talk about setting up our new idea. Ann Bennett at that time was away, so was unable to attend.

After much discussion – joy of joys – a lovely light airy room was designated to us to use as our centre. Ann and I and the Facefax team had a great time decorating and furnishing it, resulting in an extremely welcoming and peaceful area. I must thank all the people who helped to supply us with furniture, carpeting, office equipment and art work with such goodwill.

At last we were able to offer many complementary therapies, advice, legal advice, counselling and support group meetings all on a professional level, including Art Therapy which is my baby. This would be entirely run on a voluntary basis by fully qualified professional therapists and staff, and we certainly didn't have a lack of support in that area!

The room was finally ready – our dream, all those months ago, had finally materialised. A date was fixed for the official opening of the 'Dunstone Bennett Suite' as it was named, to be held on Friday 16 October 2009. We had a wonderful evening with many guests and friends attending. The Mayor of Northampton, Michael Hill and his wife Margaret, came and officially opened our new room after making a supportive and encouraging speech. Many medical members from the hospital came, and also members of the Freemasons in Northampton. We were delighted to see such a turnout and couldn't wait to start – a whole new era was about to begin. This would have been an impossible achievement without all the love, help and support we have received from so many over the years.

Very sadly, Arthur has since died, but I'm sure he would have been so proud to have seen our therapy centre grow into such an important, necessary and special place for all cancer patients. We are eternally grateful to him and to his wife Barbara for their ever constant support and encouragement.

JUST GET ON WITH IT

Looking back over my earlier years as a very young newly-wed army wife, living overseas in Aden in the South Yemen, I do believe they were quite formative years in building the foundation for facing many challenges yet to come in my life.

I learned very quickly how to cope and survive many difficult and sometimes dangerous and frightening situations. This was an active overseas posting and the Radfan War was then in full swing. It's strange what life throws at us and so often we fail to recognise at the time the importance of what's happening. Only in hindsight can we see a clearer picture.

17

I was so far from home and out of touch with all that was going on at home. There were no mobile phones, no phone to phone home to, only telegrams, but most important of all – letters. So precious and treasured by me, as I was dreadfully homesick. However, I believe this all helped to make me grow up and stand on my own feet, especially helpful when years later I faced a painful divorce. Bringing up my young children was certainly a challenge for me, but so rewarding.

I think within our family, especially my parents, our stubbornness and stoicism can be recognised in facing up to what is dished out at times. When I faced cancer many years later, I was determined to get through it – just as it came, just get on with it!

It is strange looking back over the years, because before I married, I was a rebellious art student in the early sixties. Nothing could be further removed from army life overseas to the life I had before in the heady swinging sixties.

Moving on many years later, through mutual friends, I met Brian or Bunny as he is known now my second husband. Coincidentally, we had known each other many years ago, studying art at the same college. When I was diagnosed in 1998 with cancer of the soft tissue of the mouth, it was he, my dear husband, who held me up, supported me, talked me through it and in every way battled his way with me from beginning to end, whilst I raged against the diagnosis.

Without his enduring love, I don't think I could have made it – certainly not as well as I have. I believe that the love and support he and my family and friends gave me is paramount to the rapid recovery I made. This, in turn, is what we try to do at the DB: to help and support, which is so desperately important in the painful journey of diagnosis through to recovery. There are many people who have cancer who have no one to turn to at all, hence the high suicide rates. We try to help them back on their feet again, back to a life again. No one should face cancer on their own.

We have had much feedback in so many ways from the people who have come to visit our centre. They arrive quite often worried, in pain, tired and upset, and its so very rewarding to see the encouraging results after just a few treatments from the therapies they have received.

What a long way that little acorn (a tiny idea) has grown, now becoming a young strong oak tree! Such a big thank you to all those who have helped to make it so, which is so many of you, including Becky who has raised money for us by holding various functions. Becky has come to us on a regular basis with her father, Alan, supporting him through his illness. We are eternally grateful to all those who have helped us on the way. We couldn't possibly continue without them.

A Few Problems

Earlier in my story, I have mentioned that eating in public can be quite a challenge. Fortunately for me I can still taste my food and really enjoy it apart from developing a rather sweet tooth! Whenever we are invited out, I find it easy enough with friends, but occasionally I will find myself in a situation where no one else knows or realises my predicament (swallowing is not easy.)

Do I tell them or not?

In a crowded, noisy room, it is extremely difficult to make myself heard anyway. My voice tone is now very much lower and I cannot shout. I need a quiet room to be heard. If I do try to speak up, I invariably lose my voice, which is so frustrating for me as so often I'm dying to say more and involve myself in the conversations that are going on. Usually a bended ear towards me will suffice and I can whisper into it. This can become quite an intimate affair – really amusing, depending on who it is of course! Many will say quite kindly that they are deaf anyway. I know that when someone nods at me in a puzzled and baffled way that they have totally misunderstood me. What an earth do they think I have said! Help!

One of the main problems when eating out is the amount of food delivered on my plate. I look at it often in disbelief; how can I possibly eat that much? I can't and I don't, but "eat up and clean your plate" still echoes in my memories from early childhood. If a member of my family or a close friend is nearby, they quite often remove some of the food off my plate for themselves. I have noted disbelief and horror on the faces of others at such an outrageous attack on my food, but I am really quite grateful for this. For me it saves embarrassment and I have "eaten all my food up"! I do actually eat very well and seem to maintain a fairly healthy weight balance, including the use of fortisips to top me up at times.

I did have a bit of an incident quite recently at a friend's lunch party. We had all enjoyed a wonderful meal and feeling more than a little confident, the wine helping, I decided to try some rather delicious goats cheese. This cheese proved to be an absolute disaster and trying hard to swallow, it became a nightmare. The cheese had become firmly wedged like a sponge, coating my throat, and I just couldn't shift it. Alarmingly, I began to have difficulty in breathing. Friends jumped up, thwacking me on the back, confusedly trying to advise each other in their consternation, whilst I was literally struggling not to allow hysteria to overcome me. I coughed and coughed – nothing. Suddenly a hot drink was thrust into my hands and amazingly as I swallowed, the heat helped to melt the cheese a little. At last I could breathe again, but the damned cheese was still there. Without this becoming a boring saga, it eventually shifted, but the final outcome was I had no voice at all. In fact, my voice only returned later the next day. Let this be a lesson for me as I should have known better. Honey does exactly the same thing to me, but sometimes my eyes are bigger than my tummy!

Other foods can also be a problem, for instance carrots, lettuce and rice, as no doubt many others who have had mouth and throat surgery will understand. I do find mashed potato and sauces or gravy help, as they act as a carrier. There is more information on this in the chapter for food tips and recipes.

Pronouncing words can cause problems as I have discussed earlier. This can occur not only with strangers, but also with my family and friends. Perhaps I should learn to be more patient and face others when speaking, not turning away whilst in mid-speech (particularly from my dear husband) at the most crucial moment. Sometimes this can result in hilarity, but sometimes misunderstandings can occur. I do get cross with myself, but I realise I'm lucky to be able to speak as well as I do.

For instance, when I called out to my husband saying "Jim the roofer is here", he just couldn't get it and very crossly said, "Why is the Verrucha free?" Aagh – it is so frustrating. Other times Ds and Gs are hard to form in a sentence and worst of all, my own name, 'Carol'. I'm so often asked to repeat my name again and it sounds like 'Arrow' or 'Barrel', hence my naughty sister, Judy, calling me 'Carol the Barrel'! I'm not a barrel actually I hasten to add! In fact, I'm very proud to be the 'Cover Girl' for a 'Boughton Belles' calendar, which we produced in 2004 in the village for the Cynthia Spencer Hospice, when we raised twenty six thousand pounds.

Another problem I have with post-op surgery is that my neck and shoulder stiffen up almost daily. This can be quite trying, especially when I'm doing the ironing, painting or indeed writing as I am now. A gentle massage is a wonderful way to relieve the tension, but sometimes I do require more specialised treatment.

If I am tired, and especially if my face gets very cold, I cannot speak audibly at all. It's literally a numbing experience, but at least I understand what's happening to me. I'm sure others who have similar experiences of this will sympathise, but here I am and I'm so lucky I am here and able to rejoice in life. The fact that I still have scars on my neck and arm doesn't worry me a bit. I wear my scars with pride.

However, I did have a bad experience which occurred not long ago last Christmas. Whilst parking my car in Northampton, I was confronted by a very aggressive man. He assumed I was drunk because of my speech (I was cold) and shouted to all those passing by that I wasn't fit to drive my car. It was an upsetting scene and I really wish I could have given him a piece of my mind. Too much ignorance abounds, I'm afraid, in situations such as this.

WEDDINGS

During my post-op years, we have enjoyed many weddings and were fortunate to travel to Italy twice, two years in succession, to exactly the same destination – a beautiful castle, Castello de Modanello, perched high on a hill overlooking the lovely rolling landscape of Tuscany, not far from Sienna.

On the first occasion, after a week of wedding celebrations, we spent the second week with my cousins, Karen and Stan, enjoying the delights of Rome. Many years ago Bunny had spent two years in Rome as a post-graduate art student, having won the Prix de Rome scholarship for sculpture. He proudly and knowledgeably gave us an extremely interesting guide around this magical old city. I loved it and long to return one day.

The second occasion was for Duncan, my nephew, and his new bride Islays' wedding. We were joined by all the family and many friends, including my family, Alastair and Vanessa, Clare and Connor and James and Melissa. James and Melissa had flown over especially from Canada. It was a wonderful celebration and much treasured, as family gatherings are not too frequent these days, due to everyone being so scattered about.

Duncan's beautiful wife, Islay, was diagnosed with an aggressive type of cancer a few years later while pregnant with her second child. She bravely battled her way through her pregnancy whilst receiving treatment and now has recovered and is well enough to enjoy her two lovely sons, even though she is still undergoing some chemotherapy treatment at the moment.

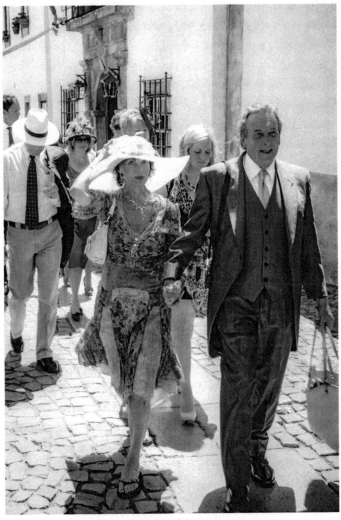

Carol and Bunny

Catching Up

The DB quickly became established at the Cripps Centre. We were gaining much support and awareness locally and with the assistance of the dedicated and happy team of professional therapists and receptionists, we found ourselves moving from strength to strength. Cancer patients and their families and carers were coming to visit us on a regular basis, supporting our belief in the work we had first envisaged and to help those who on their journey had been affected by cancer. We were thrilled to celebrate our first anniversary, toasting many more years to follow.

During this time, we were approached by David Harrop, who was then acting President of the Northampton Rotary Club. He very kindly sponsored us as his chosen charity during his year of office, presenting us with a handsome cheque at the end of the year. This support enables us to continue our work, which is all run entirely on a voluntary basis. Our local Waitrose branch, who support local community matters, also presented us with a very welcome donation.

Most importantly, I must mention Judy Shephard, my sister, who, having been elected Chairman of the Northamptonshire County Council, nominated Facefax as one of her two chosen charities, the other being SSAFA. She actively supported us during the years 2008 until 2010, finally presenting us with the grand amount of over ten thousand pounds. We cannot thank her enough for her unfailing and energetic support. All the monies which are donated help towards much-needed hospital equipment for the maxillofacial department at Northampton General Hospital, the specialised training for members of the maxillofacial staff and the general running and maintenance costs of the DB for Cancer Patients. We have succeeded in purchasing a specialist Nasendoscopy with camera, a liquid nitrogen cannister (dry ice) and therabites (jaw wideners) amongst other items.

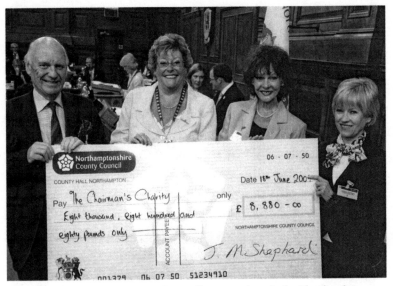

Ann and I receiving a cheque from my sister Judy Shephard

September arrived and my sister Inga and I planned a visit to Canada to stay with James, my son, and his family in Calgary. Travelling by train to Edinburgh to meet Inga, we then continued on our way to Glasgow Airport. Of course, nothing ever seems to run to plan and upon arriving at the airport, we were astounded at the news of an insurgent attack at the terminal we were flying from. Luckily we arrived after all the hue and cry had died down, but we were aghast to witness the extent of damage caused by the vehicle which had been packed with explosives and driven into the building. Quite a nerve-wracking start, but we were reassured by the amount of security which was being fully enforced following this event. We did have a wonderful holiday, but on the last day of our return, Inga had a heart problem, causing enough concern to rush her into hospital.

Fortunately she quickly recovered and was declared well enough to travel home a few days later, but I think we were both extremely relieved to get home again in one piece! Maybe the constant worry on my part of bumping into a grizzly bear in the rockies proved too much!

The following year brought about major changes with the DB. We moved to new premises in Billing Road opposite Northampton General Hospital. Here we could continue to work more independently, but still with the support from NGH, maxillofacial, oncology and Macmillan as well as GPs and dentists.

We had an official opening on 9th May 2011, and the Mayor, Marianne Taylor, declared our new rooms open. Another new start and another new adventure. We are still in Billing Road and there is more information in this book about the work we do there.

We have also had quite a lot of publicity via the media, both locally and nationally – our local newspaper, *The Chronicle and Echo*, *Image* magazine, Neon and BBC Radio Northampton are just a few. BBC Radio Northampton came to our centre to interview us all, including many of our cancer clients, highlighting the work we do.

ITV Anglia News interviewed Ann and I for an awareness campaign for Head, Neck and Mouth Cancer. This was filmed at my home and I had to prepare and cook a special soup in my kitchen whilst cameras were rolling. This was certainly a nerve-wracking experience and my hands wobbled most alarmingly. Ann and I were then interviewed about our personal experiences with cancer and a further discussion on our book, *TRILOGY*, which we had written together. It was broadcast in Anglia ITV News a few days later.

I also took part in a programme for Cancer Research UK,

which was an information film for National Awareness and Early Diagnosis Initiative (NAED). This was a series of films shown on television about early diagnosis and detection of cancer, including mouth cancer. We do try hard, but there is so much more work to do.

Even the memory of joining my good friends, Peter and his wife Jane, marching in London some years ago, supporting the Countryside Alliance, makes me realise how I could never have imagined having the strength to achieve what we have. It just shows that with a little determination and resolve – it's surprising what one can do.

A LIGHTER MOMENT

Walking every day is such an enjoyable experience for me. I walk with our dog, Percy, around the fields and lovely village where I was brought up as a child and it always brings back so many memories. It is a reflective time of the day, when I can mull over many things and mutter away to myself while putting the world to rights.

I do have amusing moments and also an adventure or two. Just recently, a very smart car pulled up alongside me and a rather good-looking young man leaned out of the window. He commented, "I rather like the look of that." Feeling enormously flattered, I tossed my head, batted my eyelashes and thanked him so much. When he enquired what breed my dog was, I realised it wasn't me he was admiring, but my dear dog! So much for vanity!

Another time, whilst walking in the fields, I noticed a strange object and picked it up. Tossing it up in the air, I proceeded to scrape the earth off it. As the object emerged in my hands, it began to look alarmingly like a hand grenade. I hastily put it down near an oak tree, making a landmark to enable me to find it again and raced home. After some excited discussion, Bunny and I called the police, who immediately alerted the Bomb Disposal Squad. The experts arrived and disarmed the grenade by blowing it up in a controlled explosion. It certainly made a big bang! Apparently, this particular field had been used as a practice area by the Home Guard during World War Two. What a fright I had and certainly not a field to walk in too often as there may well be more out there.

We also keep chickens and one day Alastair, my son, very thoughtfully presented us with two small chicks to add to our ever growing menagerie. One appeared slightly larger than the other, but we were not too concerned. However, as they grew, the brown chick called Bertha became larger and larger, sporting massive feet. And then one day I heard a sound which sounded distinctly like a crowing cockerel, albeit somewhat croaky! 'Bertha' had transformed herself into 'Bert' – a very large handsome boy and a character so colourful he deserves his own paintbox. He now rules the roost over Henny Penny, Madonna, Ethel and Madam, entertaining us with his antics. Sadly Bunny isn't quite so enamoured, especially with his gardening abilities. They are let out to roam in the garden for a few hours every day, happily wading their way through the flowerbeds and making dust baths in the borders. We still love them! Their eggs are delicious and so good for me too, as I keep telling him!

WAS THIS OUR ANNUS HORRIBILIS?

The year 2012 began quietly enough, enjoying a happy New Year's Eve with our close friends, John and Joy. We toasted good health, wealth and happiness, happily forecasting the year ahead. Little did we know what was yet to come. Was this to be our *annus horribilis*?

January began with a lovely day in London with the family, enjoying a visit to the Leonardo da Vinci exhibition. This was my brother-in-law John's birthday treat. Then, another trip to London to visit the House of Lords where we had tea, and later, with my sisters, an early evening at Westminster Cathedral. This was followed in March with a highly amusing interview with the film crew casting for the extras in the film *Les Miserables*. Needless to say, my hopes of rising to fame diminished rapidly upon seeing the vast crowds of 'young would-be hopefuls' queuing in a long snake outside the building. Great fun, though.

I was also busy working on a private commission, designing and painting ceramic tiles for a fireplace surround, and Elke my artist friend was energetically painting a huge oil portrait of me. This was something she said she had always wanted to do – very flattering for me, of course. Things were hotting up.

However, something had been niggling away at the back of my mind. Although it didn't seem too urgent a matter to address, I was beginning to allow it to overshadow my everyday life, affecting the work I was still involved with for the Facefax charity and therapy centre – although I was benefitting from much Reiki treatment.

Earlier in the autumn of 2011, I had suffered some considerable pain in my lower abdomen, resulting in an ultrasound scan to see if my appendix was the problem. I saw Mr Duncan, a consultant surgeon, who then decided to refer me to another consultant. After another scan, Bunny and I returned to see Mr Hunter, my second consultant surgeon, who explained the good news was my appendix appeared to be normal, but they had found a shadow on my left kidney; something which was a complete and total surprise. My kidney? What on earth was this about? I had hitherto felt absolutely no discomfort in the kidney region and had no other unusual signs of anything amiss. I had certainly never given my kidneys a second thought.

I was then referred to a third consultant, Mr Bell, who was a consultant urologist. An appointment was made for me to see Mr Bell at the Three Shires Hospital in Northampton. He diagnosed a tumour situated on and in my left kidney, which it was thought probably had no connection whatsoever with my former mouth cancer. A completely isolated incident.

After much discussion and more scans to follow, it was reported there was no change in the size or appearance of the left renal mass. We discussed the options of active surveillance and surgery, but I felt reassured by the results of the CT scan. Undecided whether to proceed with surgery or to continue with active surveillance, Mr Bell suggested that I took my time to consider the options, but have a repeat CT scan in six months' time. Apparently, it might well have been there for several years, and didn't appear to be a fast growing tumour. It certainly wasn't affecting my health at the time. The main concern was getting my head around this rather frightening new issue. Could I handle the time waiting whilst being monitored. What if it should grow more significantly? Kindly and well meaning family pressure was being meted out to me. Of course, they were all worried too. I tried not to think too much about it, but as time progressed, it certainly became a much heavier burden to carry. After all, this was a very silent tumour, malignant or not, and I didn't know what the hell was going on inside me. I needed to do something about it.

This niggle was growing more and more, and eventually I

made up my mind to make a new appointment to see Mr Bell. He recognised my fears and made an appointment to see Mr Potter, a consultant Urological Surgeon at Northampton. After further examinations, scans and X-rays, Mr Potter quietly suggested that an operation to remove the kidney could be arranged at Northampton General Hospital quite quickly. Thankfully, the scans revealed the tumour had not metastasised to any other organs in my body. It just appeared to be a solitary mass. Why, I do not know, but how very fortunate for me it was discovered when it was in the early stages and not when it was too late to have effective treatment. I must admit I didn't feel very brave with the diagnosis, but I knew the prognosis could be good.

A HOSPITAL EXPERIENCE

Because of all the previous surgical intervention in my throat and neck, much had to be discussed and addressed. I visited Northampton General Hospital for my pre-op assessment and was much relieved about the anaesthetic procedure I would have. Next I saw Rebecca Forster, a senior dietician at the Nutrition and Dietetic Department, and there we discussed the problems of post-op meals whilst recovering in hospital (I knew once I returned home that I could manage my own meals). I also knew that hospital meals could pose a problem for me, so it was good to know that help would be available. By this time, I was feeling fairly confident I was doing the right thing by having surgery now and not waiting any longer.

The 'day' duly arrived with a very early start in the morning. Upon arrival at the hospital, we checked in and Bunny and I were ushered into a small side room off the area for those awaiting surgery that day. With butterflies in my stomach, this was the moment of realisation. It was actually going to happen!

I had already found out as much as I could about kidney cancer and also information about the actual operation. It was hoped Mr Potter, my surgeon, would remove the entire kidney and tumour by key-hole surgery – this being far less invasive and a much faster recovery than open surgery would offer. Open surgery was only an option if inaccessibility or further complications might arise. Open surgery I hoped fervently would be a 'NO NO'!

I knew it would be very different from the surgery I had experienced with mouth cancer, but I couldn't help think 'here we go again'! At least I realised it wouldn't be so invasive, or indeed as disfiguring as surgery in and around the face and neck. However, it was still pretty serious, a major operation, and I wasn't quite sure what the outcome would be.

Various members of the medical staff popped in and out and then two anaesthetists arrived, checking me over to enormous lengths, ensuring that there would be no problems with the tubes going down my 'unusual' throat for the anaesthetic. They would both be working together and they decided to anaesthetise me via my nose and down the back of my throat, causing no further damage to my mouth. The alternative procedure risked possible tearing of the lining to the mouth and throat and damage to my teeth. I understand that due to the original surgery, my throat is now a different shape. Opening my mouth really wide is still quite problematic as I do have restricted jaw movement (I know my dentist, Jo Stock, and hygienist, Sharon Wright, will verify this).

These two delightful young anaesthetists were very kind, joking with me (I was a bag of nerves by this time), and they definitely made me feel a lot easier. I knew they would be looking after me and I would be in good hands, and with Mr Potter, my surgeon, I felt all would be well. We didn't have long to wait and suddenly the nurse and porter were ready for me. Saying goodbye to Bunny whilst being rapidly wheeled into theatre was upsetting, but once the doors closed, events happened very quickly. No time to think, nothing more, just oblivion, until I woke up.

At first in some considerable pain, I was aware of my surroundings. *Thank God, I've got through it*, I thought. *From now on, I must and will get better.* I spent a night and day in the High Dependency ward where I was absolutely astounded by the care and high level of nursing. By this time, I was aware I had received key-hole surgery – in my case, known as a laparoscopic left radical nephrectomy – and there were no other complications. Once I was able to manage my pain relief, I was moved onto the next care level in a different ward. There I became acutely aware of my vulnerability and dependency on the nursing staff in this very busy ward. I found the experience quite frightening and was very relieved when after two days I was moved again.

This ward was better and I was put in a bed in a side area with six beds, all of which were occupied, mine being the sixth bed. Here the nursing staff were friendly and caring – what a relief.

Mr Potter was pleased with my progress as I was healing up well. I had four wounds on my left tummy area and I'm sure due to all the Reiki treatment my colleagues were sending me, I was benefitting greatly from this. My main problem, yet again, was very high blood pressure, which always seems to rear its head whenever I have surgery. Another strange thing, which had occurred quite a few times earlier on in my recovery, was that whenever I opened my eyes, all I could see were my legs and feet sticking straight up into the air towards the ceiling. It took a while to understand my limbs did actually still belong to me, alarming though it was, and I realised this must be an after effect of the anaesthetic. Thankfully it didn't last for long.

The ward would become particularly busy at the weekends when many new arrivals were admitted, suffering from a rather heavy night out! Admittance of patients with mental care problems was another factor and I was greatly impressed with the nursing staff, who took time out to care and look after their special needs. I became very fond of one lovely lady who brightened up our ward, entertaining us all with her singing and dancing, sometimes donning a sick bag on her head, which doubled as a trilby hat – all delivered in a very jaunty manner.

Certainly, there was no time to be bored. I had lots of visits from friends and family, including a phone call from my son James in Canada. Soon I was well enough to go home after eight days in hospital. I just couldn't wait.

RECUPERATION

Arrangements were made for me to spend my first two nights at my sister Ingas's home, nearby in the village of Pitsford. Inga, having left Edinburgh, moved south to Northamptonshire two years before. Upon arrival, I gratefully sank into downy white sheets and pillows, relishing the sheer pure comfort – such bliss – and I slept. My son, Alastair, and his wife, Vanessa, and the grandchildren came to visit me. Libiana looked a little shocked and I realised I had lost a bit of weight! I don't think she had ever seen me ill before.

LIBIANA'S LETTER

Aged eleven years

People say it's a mirical if you survive cancer. So if once is a mirical, what do you call a twice-through cancer surviver?

34

My gran got mouth cancer in 1998—99 and had the back of her throat removed after doctors sourcing cancer there. Ever since she's always had a strong rasp as she speaks my younger sister often asks why she has an "old ladies voice". Gran has explained many times about how she must have swallowed acrylic paint (as she is an artist) and developed cancer as a result.

In 2012 she had kidney cancer. Luckily she spotted it early and had it all removed. I wasn't told at the time as I was only 9.

I would like to thank everyone, the doctors, nurses, hospitals and donators to c.r.u.k (Cancer, Research UK) for saving my Granny Gaga.

I don't know what I'd do without my Gran as she's quite a character. So yet again thank you to anyone who even donated just one penny to help save my gran and so, so many other people who have been hit by cancer.

Clare and her family arrived and it was just so lovely to see them all. I felt I was on the road to recovery.

The reason for not returning home immediately was because Percy, my beloved giant of a labradoodle, would have knocked me over in his excitement seeing me again. I had to get a little stronger first.

Unfortunately for me, Inga and Judy had previously arranged long before my hospital 'due date' to holiday north in Orkney. I was certainly not well enough to go with them. They were due to leave two days later with my cousin, Elsa, in one car with three dogs! (Elsa is kindly proofreading for me, in between writing her own book, which is an educational and brilliant Viking saga for dyslexic children). Their departure was timed for a very early hour in the morning and I kissed them goodbye.

I certainly wasn't left on my own, however. A very old school friend, Susan Blason, had driven over at the crack of dawn, whereupon she fussed over me, gave me breakfast and kept me company until Bunny arrived later on that day. I was so grateful for such kindness – what a good friend.

It was during this time that my thoughts kept returning to Sheila, another friend of longstanding. Whilst I was in hospital, Bunny had brought the devastating news of Sheila's death. She had also had cancer and tragically lost her battle, whilst I was recovering from mine. I had been feeling rather sorry for myself, but times like this can be very soul-searching. Light and shade, forever with us.

The next part of my journey was to stay with my very special friend, Claire OJ. Claire looked after me for about five days with much patience, especially as I nearly flooded her bathroom floor, enjoying my rather exuberant shower. At last, I could wash my hair! Claire fed me up, ensured I rested well, made me do some gentle exercise and generally spoiled me. I cannot thank her enough for looking after me so well.

Finally, I returned home and was joyfully met by an extremely affectionate labradoodle – never mind Bunny! Returning for a check-up with Mr Potter, I was delighted to hear the good results. The offending tumour and kidney had been successfully removed. I could continue with a normal life (well, fairly normal!) with regular check-ups every six months for the time being. Thanks heavens it was now all behind me.

THREE CHALLENGES

I had an aim now. Three things on my agenda. The first was to attend a celebration of Her Majesty The Queen's Diamond Jubilee at Burghley Park. The second was to go to a charity ball, raising money for Facefax, and the third was to be fit and well enough to travel to Portugal for a wedding. Weddings seemed to be featuring strongly already that year. We had previously attended Jim and Kay's wedding earlier in the year at Holdenby House. This was where I used to work as a ceramic artist at the start of my career. I love weddings – so full of joy and promise, and I adore dressing up as well!

Ann and I had been contacted during the winter months by Dana Hannon, who was then working as a Community Engagement Officer with Northamptonshire Link. Dana's boss, David Ward, had suggested Ann and I should represent the DB and Facefax Charity at a very important and special function at Burghley Park on 13th July 2012. This was a celebration of Her Majesty The Queen's Diamond Jubilee, a significant historical occasion with a link to the 19th Century: Queen Victoria visited Burghley House during her Jubilee year in 1897. We were invited to attend a picnic, bringing our husbands along as guests. This was very exciting and we had a wonderful day, feeling very privileged to be there. Four counties were represented, including us from Northamptonshire. I did feel extremely tired by the end of the day, but it was so worthwhile. The Queen had such a busy schedule that day, looking quite amazing. We were full of admiration for her.

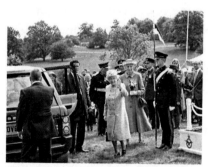

Her Majesty the Queen, Burghley Park

Next, on 7th July, came the Charity Highwayman's Masked Ball. This was organised by a very supportive and energetic group of young people in the village of Boughton. The venue was at Sywell Aerodrome in an enormous hangar, seating hundreds of guests. The ball was held in aid of three charities: The Northamptonshire Air Ambulance, Thomas's Fund and our Facefax Charity. We had a table of ten guests and Pauline Gibbings from Macmillan hosted a table next to us. It was a grand affair with an auction, entertainment and much dancing, accompanied by a delicious dinner. A huge amount of money was raised due to such hard work and effort by the team committee, and it was a great success. We were presented with a very handsome cheque donated to our Facefax Charity and we thank them very much indeed for their great support.

My third aim was to travel to Portugal and attend John and Joy's, our very dear friends, daughter's wedding. Two days after the Ball, Bunny left with John for a marathon drive from the UK to Portugal. This was to be an epic journey, and they were laden with wedding gifts, luggage and champagne for the wedding. They had a great time, taking time out for several days before reaching their destination. No questions asked here! I followed Joy a week later, flying out to Lisbon, where I was met by friends and driven to Praia Del Rey, on the coast near Obidos. There I joined company with Richard and Chris, our friends with whom we were sharing a villa near the hotel. Bunny was thoroughly immersed in wedding preparations, but joined us later. Natalie and Owain were married a few days later in a very old church in Obidos, which is a very picturesque walled medieval town, high upon a hill. It was a memorable day, adding a bit of spice with some important guests, including some members of the Royal Family.

Now thoroughly recovered from my operation and well rested, I returned home prior to Bunny's departure. The plan was that he would drive back with John, or so we thought. Never mind all my problems during the year, I'm not the only one. Bunny has had his fair share of dramas, too.

Two days later, after my return, I still hadn't heard from my nearest and dearest and was beginning to feel slightly anxious. Finally, a phone call from John, still in Portugal, explaining that Bunny was not at all well. This was worrying as no one appeared to know what was wrong. He had a high temperature and was quite delirious. He certainly wasn't fit to drive back to the UK and how they got back I dread to think, but they made it eventually.

Bunny arrived home and I just couldn't believe this apparition before me, resembling my husband. He had wasted away. The thought crossed my mind he might have suffered a stroke or even contracted Legionnaires disease. It was very scary. All this happened in such a short space of time since saying goodbye to him in Portugal, when he had looked so fit and well.

With the help of Harry, an old friend, he was rushed into the surgery, whereupon our GP diagnosed him with acute pneumonia. What a shock! To this day we do not know how this happened, but I'm so thankful he eventually recovered well enough to resume a fairly active life. It certainly knocked him for six. I don't think he had ever been so ill before in all his life. Now he treats life a little more carefully, although it took a good year to get over it.

Another Hiccup

So much for our *Annus Horribilis*, good and bad, but more was to come – this was certainly a year for ill-health. I have always struggled with the knowledge of inherent dental problems after surgery and radiotherapy treatment. One of the main factors being dry mouth – xerostomia, as its known. This is a constant trial as it affects the saliva or lack of it in the mouth and can cause gum problems, resulting in tooth decay. I am particularly aware of this and have a regular regime as I mentioned earlier in my story. I have regular check-ups at the maxillofacial department at the Northampton General Hospital where I am examined by Pamela Hall, Trust Grade Doctor in Oral & Maxillofacial Surgery, and Maxillofacial Technologists, Paul and Rob, who keep a close eye on me. A few of my teeth have caused problems over the years due to radiation treatment.

However, quite unexpectedly, whilst enjoying a summer lunch party with friends, disaster struck! I chewed on something which suddenly made my lower jaw crack. I knew immediately something was very wrong, especially as the searing pain shot up my jawbone and into my ear – all on the left side of my face, which had been affected by so much surgery. Making my excuses, I fled home only to discover the left side of my face had swollen up like a chipmunk. It was so painful and I couldn't understand the cause. I must admit I was terrified. Thankfully, I managed to make an urgent appointment the next day to see Mr Bill Smith, my maxillofacial consultant surgeon, and he examined me very carefully. He immediately arranged an X-ray of my lower face and I knew that all was not well. Mr Smith explained a few possible causes of my condition and prescribed a course of very strong antibiotics and painkillers before I was sent home.

The main worry was the onset of radio-osteonecrosis. This is when the bone in the jawbone area begins to deteriorate after a length of time following radiation treatment. I was horrified because I knew the outcome of this was pretty dire. Gradually, some of the swelling began to go down, but I was still experiencing shooting, stabbing pains in my chin and jawbone. I felt miserable and on a return visit to Mr Smith, I was prescribed another course of antibiotics. Apparently there was a possibility that the metal plate in my jawbone might have moved a little, causing pressure on the roots of my lower teeth, or even the possibility of a rogue tooth. All this was thoroughly investigated, but whatever the cause, and thank goodness it didn't appear to be radio-osteonecrosis, I ended up taking antibiotics for four months. Finally the inflammation and infection died down, leaving me feeling quite nervous, should it ever occur again. If so, I would immediately return to a prescribed course of antibiotics – wasting no time! I certainly don't relish the thought of a repeat performance.

END OF A BUSY YEAR

Later on the same year, during the month of August, my lovely niece Juliet, Inga's eldest daughter, was preparing for her marriage to Jon. An added bonus was the exciting arrival of Laura (Juliet's younger sister), who had returned from an extended grand trip overseas. The wedding ceremony took place in the city of Edinburgh, followed the next day with a wonderful reception at Ravensheugh beach, Dunbar, just outside Edinburgh. There was a huge marquee overlooking a panoramic view of the sea and sky. The weather was an absolute gift – blue skies, sunny and warm. All the family attended, including my grandchildren – apart from James and his family, who are overseas. Sadly Bunny was in the throes of recovery still and was also unable to come. In spite of my troublesome jaw, I dosed myself up and had a wonderful time. I wouldn't have missed it for the world.

Connor recalls:
I don't really have much recollection of when my granny first got cancer, although I have been told stories of how as a very young child I used to amuse her and other patients receiving radiotherapy. I suppose as I was a young and completely oblivious to what was going on around me I just carried on being the crazy and energetic child I

was. Having a granny who has had cancer twice has definitely made me more aware of the dangers surrounding cancer and has shown me how badly cancer can affect people. I am just glad that I have such a strong granny who was able to fight off that cancer not just once but twice! It truly makes me proud that she is my granny and I have so much respect for her because of it, it has also taught me that cancer is pure evil and is something I wouldn't wish on my worst enemy.

Whilst we were there, Connor, my eldest grandson enjoyed his sixteenth birthday, which reminded me of a highly energetic fourteenth birthday Judy and I had with him one summer in Orkney. We had joined him and another young friend of his on a day out on a hilly rough terrain at a Laser Zone. Dressed in full army combat, off I went ducking and diving taking pot shots at Connor and his friend – my enemy! How Judy and I survived I don't know, especially as our instructor left us to it. It was a great time, but I wouldn't do it again.

Returning home, I had a phone call from James with disturbing news. He and his family were leaving Canada and moving to Melbourne in Australia. James works for the Shell company and has been employed by them for many years, based in Calgary. This, apparently, was an opportunity not to be missed. A new challenge for us all. The length of his stay in the Antipodes was fairly uncertain. They were going to sell their home and their cars, uproot the children from school and embark on a new adventure. For them it was indeed an exciting project, but for me, I felt dismay. How and when would or could we see them all before they left for the other side of the world? Flying for me is not an easy mode of travel. How would I get to Australia? Thank goodness my fears didn't last long and I decided this could be opening up an amazing new world, not only for them, but also for me. A few days later, James phoned with the news that they would all be flying over to the UK to see us and say goodbye. They didn't have much time as they were leaving for Melbourne at the beginning of December.

James writes:

A few years after Mum and Bunny's wedding in Orkney, I moved to Canada to be closer to Melissa, my travel companion from Australia. It was in Canada where I proposed and then later married Melissa and was fortunate enough to have Mum and Bunny fly out to attend the wedding. Soon after I moved to Calgary, 'gateway to the Rocky Mountains', and have been living overseas ever since.

Keeping a family connected while living overseas has not been an easy challenge nor a foregone conclusion. I realised early on that big steps were necessary in order to keep connected with life in England and in particular Mum's on-going health. Weekly phone calls and third party updates are no substitute for flying over and spending quality time at Boughton.

So, early on in my time in Canada, I took the decision to try and return home every year or so, come credit crunch or volcanic ash. Fortunately my wife, Melissa, was fully supportive, even if my credit card grumbled otherwise. Then over time my family grew as I became a proud father to Sophie and Ben, and two visitors became four.

Mum made sure it wasn't one way traffic however. To her credit, she's never let her health situation get the better of her plans to visit Canada. Armed with as many fortisips as she could physically stuff in a suitcase, and enough bottles of water to float a battleship, she would endure the plane journey to Canada to see her grandchildren. It helped that on some occasions she was chaperoned by either Clare (my sister) and her son Connor, or with her sister Inga, but she also travelled alone, none the worse for her troubles except for the need of a stiff medicinal whiskey at the other end.

On one home visit Mum took me to the Facefax clinic at the Cripps

Centre in Northampton, to try out their Reiki therapy centre that was being offered to outpatients. Typically I am not one to volunteer for massages or spas, and as such had felt a little anxious about what to expect. I need not have worried, as it was an incredible experience that felt rejuvenating, even with the hospital photographer six inches from my face taking photos for the charity brochure!

Now that my children are getting a little older, they are able to hold conversations with their grandmother ('Gaga') much better. It's encouraging that, despite Mum's speech problems, they are still able to chat away happily together and keep the phone companies in business.

My children adore Gaga and somehow we all try to squeeze in a year's worth of catching up into a fortnight. I suppose in a way it also allows me to judge Mum's progress in a different way to my family, as our reunions are stretched out over longer spells. When Mum told me of the reappearance of cancer, where it was, and just what was being discussed to try to remove it, my worst fears were realised. I felt helpless and isolated during that period of uncertainty and leading up to the operation but again Mum confounded the odds, 'sticking it to the C-Man' and proving every battle is worth fighting.

It's now fifteen years since the initial diagnosis, and there have been some scares along the way, but it just proves what remarkable care and support my mother received, both medically and emotionally and I'm forever grateful to everyone who helped my mum succeed along that journey. She's still cracking bad jokes and forever losing her phone, so no change there!

Their visit was so precious, especially knowing what little time they had. I know Alastair and Clare and their families enjoyed the reunion very much. It was great to see their 'little Bro'! Not so little actually, as he is well over six feet tall and towers over me!

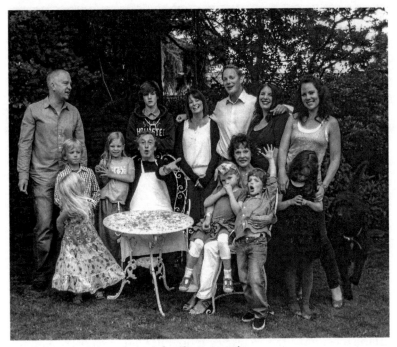

A family get-together

Autumn finally arrived and with it a dog show in the village held in the Pocket Park. With help from Julie, Eve and Jean and Ann, we set up a stand displaying information for our Facefax Charity and the DB. Judy helped with Tony's wife, Marie Boullemier, by organising a huge tombola all in aid of Facefax and they sold out in minutes! Hundreds of dogs in all varieties came with their extremely proud owners, proving to be a very successful day. Judy, Inga and I presented a special trophy; 'The Sutton Memorial Cup' for the 'Best of Show Dog'. We had this made in memory of our father, who had been a very well-known veterinary surgeon in the county. We hope the show will return next spring in 2014, as it is such a popular event.

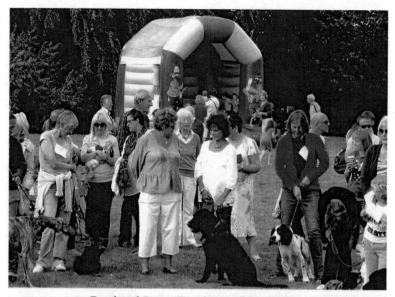

Carol and Percy, Boughton village dog show

In the meantime, the art classes at the DB Centre were continuing, along with much therapy work three days a week supporting cancer patients and carers. We decided to hold an event to raise more awareness and Ann arranged a curry evening at the Maharaja in Northampton, which was well attended.

Ann and I were yet again discussing the idea of writing a second book and with the encouragement and help from our trustees, we were excitedly sourcing a publisher. By this time, Jane Garrard, my dear friend who has stood by me through thick and thin, suggested it was time to have a well-earned break for the both of us. She was facing surgery for hip replacement and I was tired out. Off we went to Ragdale (for those who don't know – a wonderful spa), where we completely relaxed for two and half days. What better way to indulge ourselves. We do this together every year; it's our little treat to ourselves.

James and Lis had safely flown to Australia and just as we were all beginning to make preparations for Christmas, another blow. Judy's husband, John, was rushed into hospital with a suspected heart attack. He recovered well, but in the spring of the following year (2013), he underwent a quadruple heart bypass and now thankfully is doing very well – with a new spring in his step.

Out went 2012 and I think really I was quite glad to let it go. Another year ahead. What next?

SUMMERTIME

Publishing our new book was not the only criteria on our agenda for 2013. Ann and I also had to write it. Little did we realise how much work lay ahead of us, but armed with our important and urgent story and lots of enthusiasm, we embarked on our new project.

Very sadly in the early start of the year, Granny Katie passed away. Katie was my children's surrogate granny and much cherished. She almost reached the grand age of one hundred years by a few weeks. Katie had lived a happy, healthy and long life. We all miss her.

During this period, I was very involved with my ceramic art and was working on two commissions. One was a large tiled panel depicting hens and cockerels in a rural scene, to be placed behind my client's enormous Aga range. The other was a dinner service for a client who lives in South Uist in the western Isles of Scotland, and who runs a guesthouse for his fishing guests. The designs were based and sourced on the natural inhabitants of the isles: animals, birds and fish. I was having a busy time and feeling full of energy and creativity.

We had arranged a spring holiday in Cornwall and a visit to Orkney later in the summer. Bunny had celebrated his Big Birthday, having reached the 'young' age of seventy years. Ann and I had been busy giving talks to various cancer groups, and also attended a very special day at The Magdalen Centre, near Oxford. This was an invitation from Lisa Mullins, our Macmillan Regional Involvement Co-ordinator, who was organising a large discussion group concerning Macmillan Cancer Support. It was hugely supported by medical people and cancer patients from all over the country.

The work for the Facefax charity and within the Dunstone Bennett complementary therapy centre was and is increasing with the work we have achieved so far, and long may it continue.

All appeared to be going well, when one day Ann mentioned she had a problem with a tooth. She wasn't too unduly perturbed, but was going to have it checked out. The end result, as you will read in Ann's story, was quite unexpected. Ann explains in her story what next happened to her and how she coped. From my own perspective, I was completely shocked, worried and scared for her. To have cancer twice was such a blow and here was Ann now struggling yet again, with this new diagnosis. My turn last year and Ann's turn this year. Fortunately for both of us, we have managed to fight these battles and emerged into the light again. 'Onwards and sideways' as Ann often says – swimming upstream!

I think I am learning to concentrate on things I can and want to do, and not wasting time wishing for what I had or hadn't done. Every step is an arrival – at least that's what I try to think.

We have enjoyed a beautiful summer, with so much to be thankful for. I'm looking forward to next year when I hope to fly out to Australia to spend some time with my family there. In the meantime, knowing who you are and being confident in that and being happy with yourself is a mandate I endeavour to stride towards. All this can be a struggle at times, but I never try to forget that life is the greatest show on earth.

Finally, I join Ann in thanking our many friends and contributors for helping us to write and publish this book.

Chapter 3

ANN'S STORY

INTRODUCTION

It is now eight and half years since my operation for mouth cancer. This life-saving surgery involved the removal of one third of my tongue and the floor of my mouth, which was rebuilt on the right-hand side using reconstructive surgery. A piece of tissue with an artery and a vein attached was taken from my left arm – called a 'free flap' – and transplanted into my mouth to fill the gap. For anyone (not me, fortunately) with hairy arms, this is even more challenging. As Carol mentioned in her story, they then have to remove hairs from the inside of their mouth. Some lymph glands were removed on the right side of my neck. A feeding peg was inserted into my stomach, which was for me, I have to admit, very challenging. Fortunately, because I had made good progress, it was removed after five months. At this point I could manage to sustain myself by mouth, albeit with a very limited diet in terms of both the types of food that I could manage and their constituency. The other aspect I found hard to cope with was the tracheotomy. However, as a result of all this intervention, I am still alive and for that I am very grateful. This gratitude, along with keeping busy and having lots of goals both professionally and personally, are very important to both Carol and I. We stay focused on looking after ourselves as much as we can with a healthy diet and lifestyle – and have lots of fun with family and caring friends.

We wrote our first book, *TRILOGY: How to help the Mind, Body and Spirit survive Mouth, Head & Neck Cancer,* seven years ago now and looking back it has been a roller coaster of a journey with experiences taking us both up to the heights and down to the depths. You're told that after cancer, life will never be the same again – and I can vouch for that. Of course, it is an individual choice as to how one responds to the challenges. I remember one of our Facefax Trustees who'd had a similar operation around the same time as me saying what hard work it is being a survivor. To that, I would also add HIGH Maintenance, in keeping oneself fit and healthy in mind, body and spirit.

Before my own diagnosis, my sum total experience of how someone else deals with a life-threatening illness was somewhat limited. My cousin's wife, Jackie Jowett, was given three years to live after her diagnosis for cancer. Her son, Max, was nine years old at the time and her daughter, Vicky, six, so her first priority was putting her children's welfare in order. She then concentrated as best she could on living the rest of her life to the full. My father, on the other hand, three years before he died, knew he did not feel well and was told by his doctor to go away, to get his sense of humour back and to enjoy life. He did his best to follow the doctor's advice. He had no idea that he had a serious heart condition – none of us did, not even my mother. After he had died, I bumped into his doctor who told me that he knew my father had three years to live, but if he had told him, my father would have almost certainly died much sooner.

On the eve of my own operation, my sister, Sarah Erickson, said that we needed to talk about what would happen if I did not survive the nine-hour ordeal. Until that point, no one had even hinted at the fact I might not make it through. I would be lying if I denied that the possibility had crossed my own mind, though. I struggled to think about what I wanted and made a bit of a joke about it, saying to Sarah, "Buy red roses to give to friends in a big arm-expansive gesture" – for those who remember it, as if I was in a Morecambe and Wise show where a lady used to come on at the end and say 'I love you all'. I knew Sarah meant well, so I half-heartedly thought about which hymns I would like at my funeral and I can recall Michael being quite relieved that I did not want a full Requiem Mass. These days, there is an NHS publication freely available called *Planning for Your Future Care*. This is not a bad idea actually as it certainly broaches the subject, saving relatives having to figure out how to have this type of conversation when emotions are running high. More importantly, it is a prompt, putting the sufferer calmly in control of their own wishes, rather than leaving it too late. For a downloadable version of this publication, visit www.nhft.nhs.uk.

Before my cancer was diagnosed, I had undergone surgery on my back. The one condition ran on from the other and so I was pretty much incapacitated for a period of three and a half years in total. That's when I discovered how hard it is going from being a very active person to doing very little, so I tried to find a way of using my expertise as a Hypnotherapist and Reiki Practitioner to occupy me and help others at the same time. It is also why, as soon as I felt up to it, I got together with my old friend, Dr Addy Hackett. Addy is a Consultant Clinical Psychologist. We first got to know each other when we both attended a clinical hypnotherapy course in 1996. We have remained friends ever since and look forward to working together whenever we can.

Addy recalls:

> *"In 2005, whilst recovering from extensive surgery, Ann worked as a volunteer hypnotherapist at Cynthia Spencer Hospice for a few months under my supervision. She worked with some of the patients*

who were feeling stressed about their situation or about the treatments they were undergoing. Ann was extremely effective in helping patients relax and was very able in helping the staff understand those patients' needs. On one occasion, I remember Ann was conducting a session with a patient who had a well-known phobia about needles. She had quietly asked the doctor in advance that when he walked into the room he should have removed his tie, so as not to change the mood, which he willingly did. This is just one lovely example of many I have experienced, demonstrating what an empathy Ann has, understanding patients' needs and effectively communicating them to their medical team. Sometimes words are not required; her demeanour says it all."

Thank you Addy and Cynthia Spencer Hospice for having faith in me. A hospice is a truly wonderful place and I do so admire those who are able to work with the terminally ill and their families. Whilst I enjoyed my short time there, I felt it wasn't right for me. However the experience did make me want to be more proactive and it spurred me on to join the Facefax support group, hoping I might be useful. Carol originally set up the group in 2001 and she was interested in doing more at that time, too.

Carol and I were (and still are) very grateful for all the support we received from our fellow Trustees, our families and our friends, and so it was very important to us not only to launch *TRILOGY* but to have a party for all those who had helped us – which we threw in October 2006. Suzanne Linnel, a friend of mine, ran the Great North run to raise funds for us. Gary Osborne, from Ossie's on the Wellingborough Road, Northampton (a clothes shop where I am a regular customer) and his daughter, Sally, put me in touch with their friend, Keith Napier, who is a member of the Old Northamptonians' Association Rugby Football Club. He kindly asked Beverly Kevan, the clubhouse administrator, if we could hold our launch there. Beverley agreed and said there would be no charge as she felt that we were a worthwhile charity. Mark Lee was MC and did an excellent job. Ossie's put on a fashion show. Reiki Academy provided the finger buffet free of charge and my therapy friends offered complementary therapies – they were kept very busy. Barclaycard matched the raffle monies raised and we auctioned some great prizes, which had been very generously donated. It was a memorable evening helping to raise the awareness of mouth cancer; we raised funds for the Maxillofacial Clinic and sold a lot of books, the proceeds of which were donated to Facefax.

Of course, there was bubbly on arrival – which for us, did and still does represent a CELEBRATION OF LIFE. In my opinion, it is the only way to start any party. AMAZINGLY, everyone involved has agreed to do the same again. Fantastic! We are eternally grateful. Already, Suzanne has kick-started fundraising by completing the Edinburgh Marathon. If the launch of the second book is half as successful as the first, then it will all have been worthwhile. A fabulous start to proceedings, with sales rolling in and maximising the amount that can be given to the charity.

In 2007, the highlight for Carol and me was when we were on a Macmillan buddying/befriending course in London for two days. At the end of the first day, I suggested to Carol that as it was Thursday and late night shopping, we ought to go into Oxford Street's Waterstones and check if *TRILOGY* was available as we had been told it would be. Sure enough, there it was on the shelf under 'Health'. We were so excited, we could have kissed the staff. We introduced ourselves and explained why we had written our book; how we needed their help to generate sales and promote awareness because this type of cancer, even though it was rare, was on the increase especially in younger people. Indeed, seven years on, this is sadly still the case and Maxillofacial Clinicians no longer consider it to be the rare cancer it was when I had it in 2004. Needless to say, when we left Waterstones that evening, we were euphoric and promptly went across the road to St Christopher's Place for a celebratory glass of champagne (for those that don't know this easily missed courtyard, it is down a small alleyway next to Selfridges where you can sit, eat and drink, while watching the world go by).

Around this time, I lost a very close friend, Stephanie Tuckley. We had known each other for a very long time. Steve, as her friends called her, had been diagnosed with her cancer whilst I was recovering from mine. Thankfully, Steve survived and we celebrated that fact many times. Sadly, a couple of years later, she lost her battle. It's almost a hollow victory when you survive and your close friend does not. I often think of her and the fun times we had. I feel I owe it to Steve to make the most of my 'post-cancer' life and not to waste a moment.

We do feel particularly passionate about supporting young sufferers. Carol and I both know what a tough journey all cancer patients have, but when your ability to communicate changes, when your way of eating is a challenge, and your weight and body mass reduces, it is a long, long journey back to finding a new 'normal' and accepting that life will never be the same again. Visible, unsightly scars and other related issues can knock one's self-confidence hugely, even at mine and Carol's age, and so much more so for someone younger. Every time you look in the mirror, you are reminded of what you have been through. Of course for some, weight loss might be a bonus, but for me it has always been a challenge to keep weight on; I also have long-standing allergies and food intolerance problems. I happen to love my food, so I am pretty determined to source tasty alternatives.

Shortly after the launch, we had a call from Anglia TV asking us to talk on television about the book. We had very little notice. Mr Colin Harrop, my consultant, was also invited to be part of this Anglia News item, giving the medical lowdown on mouth cancer. As always, he did not hesitate to support us. One part of the interview was to be filmed in Carol's kitchen, where she would be making soup. When you have the kind of surgery that we had, soup becomes a very big part in your life. My great friend Erika Takacs still makes me soup, as she has done since day one of my journey. As I was leaving my house that day, I had a call from Carol asking me to pick up one carrot and one onion on my way. High on adrenalin and excited about the interview, I was on a mission! I flew into Smith's farm shop and demanded said veg in such a way, they must have wondered what part a carrot and an onion could possibly play in a matter of life and death.

Because I like scarves, I now rely on them to cover the scars on my neck – whilst adding a mood-enhancing splash of colour to any outfit on any occasion – and they asked if they could film me putting one on. All very well, but in the heat of the moment and being so petite, I could hardly reach the mirror and looked very awkward doing something I do every day, normally, without any effort.

The year after *TRILOGY* was published I went to The Royal College of Surgeon's Faculty of Dental Surgery in London with Anne Hicks, the maxillofacial clinical nurse specialist and our supporter, to give a talk on the patient's perspective on having mouth cancer – with a copy of *TRILOGY* under one arm, of course. I had been made aware after one of my earlier talks that the medical profession can sometimes forget the patient and underrate what the patient is going through – having too much focus on science, medical matters and finance, which clearly do play a large part. I am pleased to say the consultants that I have seen have never made me feel like that. It was daunting to face such a prestigious audience, but I felt it was important to do it, nonetheless. The feedback I received was so uplifting. One of the comments from a medical professional actually said, "How very useful, hearing an in-depth view from the other side of the fence." We also sold quite a few more books as a result.

A similar instance I recall was when Dr John Aherne, senior partner at Weaver's Medical Centre in Kettering, and his wife came to the DB for John to have Reiki, which we usually recommend to patients who are having treatment for cancer. Dr Aherne has since died, but I am telling this story with Mrs Aherne's permission. In my capacity as a Facefax and DB Trustee, I am often requested to listen and chat to clients and their supporters, and that day John asked me to explain my role. One of the topics John and I discussed was the delivery of 'bad news'. Unfortunately at the DB we do hear complaints from distressed clients and we endeavour to help those individuals look at their diagnosis in a more positive light, helping them come to terms with the situation and helping them to have reasonable goals designed to encourage them not to give up before their time. This is where my own experience with cancer, coupled with helping cancer patients through my own hypnotherapy and Reiki practice, stands me in good stead, I feel.

John was very interested in all that the DB stood for and as a result of our discussions, he invited me to give a talk to a GP group at the Woodlands Private Hospital near Kettering. This talk was not only to promote the services of the DB, but also the importance of how the medical professional delivers the cancer diagnosis. Anne Hicks came with me to answer the medical questions and once again our talk was considered to be thought-provoking. Mission accomplished! It was not long after this talk that John sadly passed away. I only had a short time to get to know this lovely man and his lively wife Liz and I will always be grateful for the support he, as a GP, gave to the DB and the work it does.

Michael and I, after I had recovered from my operation, decided to build ourselves a house. For us, this meant living on-site in a caravan for eleven months through the coldest winter for fifty years. Another challenge I surprised everyone by rising to! Proof of my belief that if you survive major life-saving surgery, things just don't faze you in the way they might have previously. That winter it was so cold, we needed to put hay all the way round the outside and underneath the caravan for extra insulation. When I looked out first thing each morning, I felt I was in a manger, which just before Christmas, was truly apt. I was really in the spirit of the season!

One night whilst living there, I had left Michael childminding, having decided to come home by myself for an early night. It was just after midnight. I was asleep in the caravan alone when I was awoken by a flashing torchlight at the bedroom window. Aware that someone was outside, I rang Michael to see if it was him. Having established it was not and whilst still speaking to him very quietly on the phone, I crept along to the other end of the caravan where there was a big picture window to see if I could see who it was. I was standing quite close by when whoever was out there threw something at the window and within seconds, there was a second thud and shattered glass everywhere.

Much to my astonishment, I let out a very loud scream, followed by me shouting, "The police have been called. Get out!" I ran back to the bedroom, shaking. I heard Michael saying that he had, in fact, called the police who were on their way. Even though this was all going on, the biggest shock of all was that I had been able to scream and shout, projecting my voice in such an effective way. It must have been the adrenalin, because under normal circumstances, even when having an argument with Michael for instance – we can be quite feisty with each other – my voice really struggles to do justice to my side of the argument.

Years before, we had been victims of a peeping Tom, and even when I'd seen him and wanted to attract Michael's attention, I opened my mouth to shout but nothing came out. Actually, I need not have worried because when Michael did realise I was trying to tell him something, he flew out of the house, sounding like Tarzan, and chased him away. MY HERO!

INDIA

Those of you who read our first book will be aware that my husband Michael was born in DehraDun, India; his family being fourth generation British Army, dating back to the time when Colonialism ruled. The need to revisit his birthplace became important to Michael, as he was only three years old when he left on a ship to Australia with his mother and siblings.

Three years after my operation, we decided to go there with my cousin David and his wife Lesley. David, like Michael, is ex-military and was very interested in visiting the Army Officer Academy in DehraDun.

Michael planned where he wanted to visit, which meant a good bit of travelling, from the foothills of the Himalayas right down to Kerala in the South West region of India. A private travel company took over Michael's itinerary and booked a driver/guide, together with the fourteen hotels that we would need over the three weeks.

I was well aware that a visit to India would be an education and I was a little apprehensive about my first trip there to say the least. My friends expressed concern that our visit was not always going to be within my comfort zone – not even close to it. After all, this was not going to be the typical trip enjoyed by so many Europeans staying in five and six star hotels, travelling around the Triangle of wonderful cultural sites and palaces – although we did incorporate all of these in our itinerary.

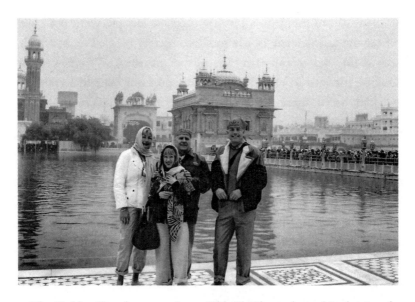

The Golden Temple, a prominent Sikh Gurdwara located in the city of Amritsar, Punjab, in the North Western part of India. We had to remove our shoes. Even though it was cold, we took off our socks too, to keep them dry, as the paths were wet. L-R Lesley, Ann, Michael, David

As you know by now, I love a challenge and I would always have regretted not rising to this one. When you have experienced mouth cancer and all it incorporates, you feel you can face anything. As it turned out, our trip could have warranted a book all of its own; to give you an insight, of the fourteen hotels we stayed in, seven were good and the rest – well, I don't think they held any stars at all, ever!

Diet and amenities were certainly very difficult at times, but my main concern was hygiene. I packed bottles of Tea Tree oil and used it on planes, boats, trains and even on a beach! I insisted that all four of us used it and was continually soaking paper hankies so we could all regularly inhale the natural antiseptic. The rest of the passengers had no choice but to inhale it, too. For me, it was a priority, not to mention a bit of a giggle as people were not sure where the unexpected aroma was coming from. The beach, which was at the end of our trip, was not so amusing. We were really looking forward to enjoying this last lap of our tour in Kerala, as we had heard there were some beautiful beaches and tropical vegetation there. Unfortunately, the reality for us was that the hotel we were staying in was surrounded by poverty and squalor: the locals, as always, were smiling and accepting of their lot. The beautiful beach I was expecting was not beautiful at all, but covered in refuse. Not wishing to be contentious, but in this case, I do blame the authorities. I have never walked on a beach, even in equally poor countries, and had to cover my mouth with a hanky dowsed in tea tree oil because of the stench of rotting animal carcasses and human excrement. Unfortunately, it was the only way to get to where we needed to be.

I did contract 'Delhi Belly', as did Michael, even though generally he has the constitution of an ox. In my case, I put it down to a cup of coffee I had in the foothills of the Himalayas, which may not have been made with boiled water. Incidentally, the others had Chai, a milky boiled sweet tea served very hot, which Lesley and David loved and continued to enjoy throughout the three weeks.

The food was always going to be a difficulty for me, being hot and spicy – after all, this was India. It smelt delicious but not at all good to eat for people who have had oral surgery, as the lining of the mouth becomes sensitive and sore and the consequence of lack of saliva glands in the area leads to increased aggravation. As you might imagine, I did lose weight, which I could ill afford, because existing on rice, vegetables and corn flour/gram flour chappati was the only answer – and not a major issue really as it was only for three weeks.

I am very lucky where I live in Northampton. As curries do not always have to be hot, I was determined after my mouth cancer to find a way around the problem. Both the MAHA-RAJ-A along the Wellingborough Road and the Spice Indian restaurant in Duston kindly cater especially for me with a very mild curry made with coconut milk. Thankfully, I can continue to enjoy the wonderful flavours and spices found in curry, without the chilli-induced heat and resulting discomfort.

Touring Delhi in a rickshaw was the scariest of experiences. It brought to mind the television series in March of last year called *The Toughest Place To Be*. In one episode, a London taxi driver was temporarily relocated to do his job in Mumbai. After some training on the roads and in the geography of the area, he mastered it. Even as a professional driver, he found it pretty frightening at times. I now know why. If it's not a cow walking in front of you, it is a lorry heading straight for you on your side of the road. Woe betide you if you are in the way of either.

Our guide Ved, an educated and good-looking young man, wanted to take us to his family home where his father was the owner of most, if not all, of the village. We did not expect it all to be so very simple. In fact, it was quite biblical and we felt so humbled that we were moved to the point of tears. Ved had advised us to take sweets for the children, which we did. David handed them out and immediately became the Pied Piper with what seemed to be one hundred children dancing around him. I was asked by two boys who were around my height which school I went to and if I was twelve years old! I know I am not very tall, but really! As you can imagine, I lived off this tale for the remainder of the holiday and often used it to my advantage.

When we got to Dehradun, David temporarily became our spokesperson, for when Michael was so very moved by returning to his birthplace that he temporarily lost the ability to speak. We were so looking forward to taking tea with the commanding officer, who was also going to show us around – so much so that Lesley and I had brought special outfits from England to wear. Unfortunately, however, the previous night was spent in a damp and cold summer palace in a hill station called Mussoorie, known for its 'naughty goings-on' during the Colonial years. The views overlooking the Himalayan ranges were fantastic, but we had very little sleep, no hot water to wash in and damp horsehair blankets to sleep under. We just about mustered enough energy to look presentable. This was not our idea of being English ladies in what had been Colonial India years ago. Sadly our dresses returned home, unworn!

To summarise, we remember our holiday as a true reality check. We each have our own daunting and sometimes funny stories to tell, but we all agree how sobering it was to witness people in such dire conditions still smiling. Of course, there is another side to India which is beautiful and rich, as our Asian friends in the UK will confirm, and those who can afford to give generously to charities. Clearly the problems are so colossal, much more needs to be done and on a far bigger scale.

In conclusion, India, like Africa, made me think deeply at times. Whilst both are poor in places, I find Africa raw, deep and full of soul. India, before I had been there, had the reputation of being a spiritual country, but in retrospect I realise this is far too superficial and simple a description. Certainly in their own ways, both countries are fascinating, unforgettable and, for me, unmissable. What's more, they remind me to count my blessings and remember how 'lucky' I am to have fought my battle against mouth cancer here in the UK.

Out Of Africa

I have travelled to South Africa on numerous occasions. My sister, Sarah, and her husband, Charles Erickson, used to live there and since our dear friend, Trudie, emigrated from the UK to the Cape, we have visited her and her family many times. Three years ago, she retired with her partner, Tom, to a private game reserve just outside the Kruger National Park, where they built a traditional bush lodge. They have all the luxury of modern living, but are set deep in the reserve and on the bank of the Sandspruit River, where game roams freely! A visit there was timely for Michael and I to explore that part of Africa from a non-tourist point of view and it brought about a special bond between body and soul, especially after what I had been through. Being close up and at one with nature is hard to describe unless you have been there, done it, felt it, and soaked up the experience of the Bush. I have always maintained that Michael, in his safari hat, khaki bush clothes and sun tan, looks more at home than in the UK and if I didn't put my foot down, he would be bashing through the undergrowth, searching for rhino, wild dog, elephant, warring tribes and sea! You can tame a man after forty years of marriage, but the adventurer is never far beneath the surface!

Most days around five-ish in the afternoon, as the heat of the day subsides, when in the UK people are getting ready to finish their day's work, Trudie and Tom pack up their game vehicle with food and wine and head out for a daily game drive. At the furthest point from home, they unpack by a tranquil dam, watch the hippos displaying their very large mouths and, with sundowners in hand, enjoy the spectacle of the sun setting behind the mountains.

We were on a drive with them one particular evening and had stopped for sundowners, knowing that rain was imminent. As we relaxed, you could tell from the sounds that the animals – and their predators – were just beginning their nightly activities. All of a sudden, it started to pelt down, so we jumped back in the open-topped game vehicle and headed for the shelter of home, several miles away via dirt roads. Next thing we knew, the vehicle was deep in mud, and in the poor visibility, what we thought were boulders in the road ahead, turned out to be three huge rhino huddled together. I cannot describe the ADRENALIN RUSH! The sight of these magnificent animals, emerging through the pouring rain, thunder and lightning was spectacular – and just yards from us! Finding our way home in those conditions was far from uneventful – our next encounter was a herd of buffalo, who, just like the rhino, were more interested in sheltering close together than charging at the six people who were also trying to protect themselves from the elements. Back at the lodge, we were met by the staff who seemed bemused by our near-hysterical state, brought about by our potentially dangerous encounters. Laughter is a great stress buster, as Carol and I have found on many occasions. It certainly helps to be blessed with a sense of humour.

As you can see from this photograph, taken on our return that evening, we are soaked to the skin – note mine and Trudie's running mascara!

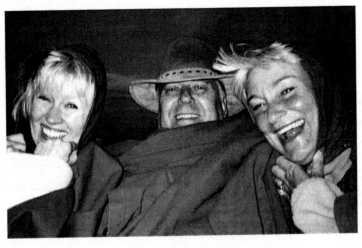

It is important to remember that on game drives, you are perfectly safe when looking into the eyes of a lioness standing six feet away, as long as you do not break the outline of the vehicle by standing up or speaking loudly.

At night in the Bush, you can't help but listen to the sounds of the animals. At times it gets so loud and goes on for so long, you wish there was an 'off switch' so you could get some sleep. When the screeching gets so loud and it is clear that something is fighting for its life, I wrestle with the local tale that impala – with the 'M of McDonalds' displayed so clearly on their rear end – are the 'fast food' of the Bush with virtually every other animal being their predators. Poor things. In the darkness, their vulnerability played on my mind, and I recalled my own apprehension and how vulnerable I felt when on a previous visit I had been invited to take part in a walking safari. I'd thought about it for a while but then chose to 'go for it'. Out in the Bush, we were told to walk behind the chief tracker in a single file: any snakes in our path would flee sideways from the vibration of footsteps and so we would be safer than if we were walking abreast and risking treading on them, or worse, them shooting up our trouser leg! Distracted by these thoughts, I suddenly found myself away from the main group. Filled with trepidation, I soon caught up. That night, I had a dream in which I was the lone impala who became separated from the herd and was picked out by a lion. As soon as it pounced on me, the impala became unconscious, so I did not actually experience any of the horror of being attacked and killed. Since then, rightly or wrongly, my belief is that the animal goes into shock and is not aware of what has happened. I could still never bring myself to watch 'a kill' but I no longer worry about the victim's suffering in the same way. Clearly, the walking safari experience and subsequent dream that night served a useful purpose for me!

As a surprise one day, Trudie had used her considerable influence to book us in for some therapeutic treatments at Elton John's favourite bush lodge, which happened to be nearby. The surroundings were fantastic and we were really looking forward to the TLC. I cannot remember the name of the lovely girl who was my masseuse, but after answering 'yes' to the consultation question, 'have you had cancer?' she asked me about my medication. I told her I was not taking any. She then proceeded to massage my back just like Kay Hughes back at home. To my horror, this girl proceeded to tell me that she was being treated for bone cancer and was in pain. I asked her what on earth was she doing giving treatments in her condition. She told me she had no health insurance and that she needed the money for her medication. My heart went out to her and I immediately embraced her. Stories like hers are a reminder that we are so lucky here in the UK to have the NHS.

The next day, we flew to Johannesburg on our way to the Cape. I was worried as my tongue and mouth were becoming very sore. I was trying to keep it to myself, but back in civilisation, I decided that a trip to a walk-in clinic in Santon was important. As luck would have it, the doctor I saw there was a specialist in mouth cancer. I could not believe it. After checking me out, he suggested it was the malaria tablets which I had been advised to take back in the UK that had been causing the inflammation and advised me to stop taking them immediately. Over the next few days, everything settled in my mouth. What a relief.

The last leg of our journey we spent in the Cape with Trudie's children, Matthew, my goddaughter Charlotte and their father Mike. It is always lovely to see them as we have known the children all their lives. Whilst there, tragically a member of Trudie's staff from her 'country guesthouse' days had lost her baby. Trudie and I attended the funeral, which as you can imagine was moving and emotionally draining. However, when Frexchia spotted Trudie and me amongst the mourners, she stopped, threw her arms around me and asked how I was (she had heard about my cancer from Trudie). I was totally taken aback by how this poor girl, grieving for her own lost child, could possibly think of anything or anyone else – but she did, and her generosity of heart and spirit is something I will never forget.

I have met some fascinating, lovely people in South Africa and Michael and I have always enjoyed the rich diversity of the country. Like the UK, they have their problems, but to my mind, Africa, once in the blood, is like a magnet to the heart and has great depth of soul. Experience it if you can …

Thank you Trudie for looking after Michael and I so well in Africa. You have always been very generous and you have given us such wonderful memories, which we will treasure for the rest of our lives.

ON A MISSION IN NEW YORK

I love New York – so vibrant and diverse. The city that never sleeps. When I was invited to join Yvonne Miller and my goddaughter, Fern, for a five-day trip there, I jumped at the chance. My previous trip with Michael had been a bit of a haze. We had tried to do it all in three days, whilst suffering from jet lag on our way home from Hawaii.

Second time around, we had a great time – listening to Gospel singers on a Sunday morning at B.B. King's Blues Club, sipping cocktails in the Marriott's "Revolving Skyline" Cocktail Bar on Broadway, not to mention some interesting cultural visits. Fern, who was seventeen years old at the time, had great fun in Time Square with the patrolling NY Cops.

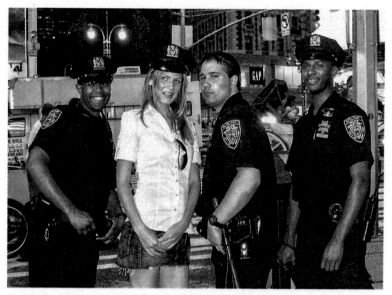

Fern in Times Square

When out and about, and left to our own devices, there is no telling where Yvonne and I will end up. Let's just say on one day out, we set off to go to Ellis Island to see the Statue of Liberty but ended upon the wrong boat, going to Long Island instead. We did see the Statue of Liberty, but from across the water! On the fifth day, Yvonne and Fern went sightseeing and we arranged to meet up in Central Park later in the day.

I went to visit the New York Memorial Sloan-Kettering Cancer Center, which boasts more than 400 physicians specialising in cancer. My New York taxi driver poured his heart out to me regarding the state of his personal life. Quite honestly, it was difficult to concentrate because of the many distractions going on outside the cab, but I don't think he noticed!

I felt very small in such a large building with an atmosphere that was totally electric, full of very busy people including very smart security men. I was on a mission, so they weren't going to faze me. Having taken directions, which meant a lift for several floors, I eventually reached the Head, Neck and Mouth cancer ward armed with a copy of our first book, *TRILOGY* (which had been published with Author House in America and still selling). I was warmly received. They were interested in the book, especially when I told them I had been a mouth cancer patient myself. They took the copy from me to put into their library, along with the order details for anybody interested.

From there, I went to Barnes and Noble – the equivalent to our Waterstones – to check if our book was available and to introduce myself. While waiting there, I got chatting to the receptionist who told me about a walk-in cancer centre in the city, which had been set up with charity money and was run by volunteer professionals. It opened once a week to patients and their carers, offering a wide range of treatments. I was immediately interested because Anne Hicks, Carol, Christine Gould and myself had talked about opening exactly that kind of centre here, but it had just remained on our wish list. This got my head buzzing with ideas and when we returned, I suggested to Carol that we started fundraising for a centre to help all types of cancer patients and their supporters and see if people embraced the idea. It proved to be a great success and although we had a lot more money to raise, we believed with the help of our friends and contacts that one day this dream might become a reality. Just eighteen months later, the DB opened its doors.

THE DUNSTONE BENNETT COMPLEMENTARY CENTRE

The ethos of the DB is to take a positive approach at a very challenging time of life. This positivity can, as it has in many cases, lead to a client's life being extended and some quality brought back at a time when this almost seems an impossibility, both for the sufferer and for their families. At the DB, we prefer to use the term 'client' rather than 'patient' because we feel this helps to keep the individual moving along on their journey. At the DB, we work closely with medical professionals and MacMillan, and indeed 95% of our referrals come from these sources. We never promise a cure, just support and understanding.

Following my operation, it took me four more years to fully appreciate how important support for carers and families is. Carol and her sister Judy Shephard had arranged a barn dance. When Michael returned the obligatory champagne flutes, he was casually asked by the staff if the party had been a success. Apparently, when explaining that the event had been in support of his wife's charity Facefax, he had burst into tears, right there, in the shop. Up until this time my strong husband, who had been fantastic support to me over the four years, had never expressed his own feelings – to the extent that sometimes I wondered if he really felt anything very deeply. To think he had bottled up his emotions all that time and I had not been able to help him access them really saddened me.

Cancer touches practically every family I know, directly or indirectly. When the sales director of our company, Eugene Murray, was told that his father – also called Eugene – had a brain tumour, he brought his father to see me and I explained to him about the DB and what it could offer him in terms of support and advice. After more talking and some Reiki from me at home, Eugene's father felt more positive about his situation and agreed to come to the DB the following day. The DB now helps sustain him and despite his original diagnosis, Eugene senior has just celebrated a significant birthday. We were touched that, at their party, his family chose to raise money for the DB as a 'thank you'.

I remember one evening taking a call inviting Carol and I to a fundraiser on behalf of Disney Ward, the children's cancer ward at

Northampton General Hospital (NGH). Sadly, we were unable to go, but once in my mind, I could not stop thinking about the children with cancer and their families. This led me to discuss with Carol and Anne Hicks the possibility of the DB offering its services to the families of the Disney Ward outpatients. We worked out a proposal, which we put to Clare Stockley and Jane Tebbutt, Disney's Paediatric MacMillan Lead Specialist Nurses at the time. They welcomed our ideas and agreed to a six months' trial period of us talking and listening to the parents and their children at Disney Outpatients on Wednesday afternoons. Christine Gould, who has both therapy skills and had been a teacher, joined me in the project. She was marvellous with the children, drawing and being creative with them whilst they were waiting for their treatments, whilst I talked to their parents about how the DB could help them – by, amongst other things, encouraging them to take a little time for themselves. This also included listening to how supporting a child with cancer had impacted their lives. Our role was designed to help divert thoughts away from the treatment their child was about to undergo, and, for a moment, help them consider how important their feelings were in a world where their children's wellbeing was generally everyone's uppermost consideration. We selected four therapist volunteers from the DB who were interested in working at Disney and who, together, offered the appropriate range of skills and had previous experience in working with children in a medical environment.

Although we were already security checked for our DB work (thirty-two of us very generously paid for by Alderwood), we six had to get DBS (previously CRB) checked to work with youngsters and vulnerable adults, and also be officially classified as NGH volunteers through the hospital human resources department as well.

Shortly before we started our Disney project, The Maha-raj-a

Indian Restaurant in the Wellingborough Road, Northampton, offered to host a PR evening for us to announce that Facefax and the DB were extending their services to children with cancer and their families. We invited Dr Vindi Koodiyedath and Dr Ali, both consultant paediatricians. Dr Ali gave a talk about their work, pointing out that children with cancer are often remarkably resilient, and highlighting the wonderful support already offered by Disney Ward and Disney Outpatients. It was clear from what he said that it was the parents and siblings who struggled the most with the worry of the illness and the strain of how the treatment would affect their loved one. As I listened, my thoughts were transported back thirty years to when my cousin's wife Jackie died of cancer when her two children were aged nine and twelve. As their father, Derek, was already in his late sixties, it had been agreed with their mother that Michael and I would be there to help him to look after them and indeed, if anything happened to him whilst the children were growing up, we would become their guardians. Nowadays, there are charities such as Kidsaide to support children through such crises. If such help existed then, we were unaware of it. At the time we were in our early thirties, with one child of our own, and were not at all knowledgeable about the trauma that cancer could cause in a family, so we muddled through and did our best. Thankfully, Derek survived until his children, Vicky and Max, became adult. He has since died. We all remain very close, as do Vicky's husband, Oscar, and their two lively boys, Andrew, aged eight, and Benjamin, six, and Max's partner, Rumi.

As I write, I feel at one with the way the DB's services have developed and been humbled by the wonderful support given by all the volunteers. Carol and I are so proud of them. Each and every one of them give from their heart. Through their efforts, we are continually, and relentlessly, raising awareness about the Facefax

Charity and the benefits the complementary therapies dispensed at the DB can have. The centre has evolved to treat all types of cancer and support for their carers, and now extends to Disney outpatients.

A FEW PROBLEMS TO OVERCOME

In the last three years, I have had check-ups every six months because I get soreness and ulcers in my mouth. I have suffered from these for many years and the condition is aggravated by certain foods. It's called Lichen Planus of the mouth and affects the skin and lining. It is quite common and found in approximately 2% of men and women in the UK, and is more common in people over forty years old. I was in my mid-thirties when it first occurred, following a fall on my back. Maybe the shock of that brought it on, who knows! The cause is unknown – not cancer, nor an infection – but it is believed to be related to the immune system. Two years ago, I had a biopsy to confirm the condition. For me, it can be difficult sometimes not to think it is something more sinister. I am grateful therefore that Mr Harrop checks my mouth twice a year and the Hygienist, Sharon Wright, every three months. I manage my symptoms with recommended mouthwashes and with Gengigel to rub onto the inflammation.

Another of my challenges is Xerostomia, which means dry mouth, caused by the absence or diminished quantity of saliva brought about as a result of surgery – in my case, eight years ago. Xerotin spray is a saliva replacement, which I use to moisten my mouth when it becomes dry. I always carry it in my handbag and I use it regularly at night. Again, as with Lichen Planus, anything acidic or spicy aggravates the problem. A tip I picked up when I attended a Hypnotherapy AGM in London on how to solve a dry mouth, in any given situation, was to imagine sucking a lemon. Trust me, it works. The trouble is, I don't often remember to do it.

The other problem is choking when swallowing, which can become very embarrassing especially if I am at a dinner party or in a restaurant. This is one of the reasons why it takes me so long to eat. To calm me down and help me not panic, I use Self Hypnosis. Hypnotherapy and Self Hypnosis are wonderful tools to help with so many different situations. I use the techniques a lot, especially if I wake up in the night and start worrying about something. It is easier for me, having had good tutors and training. That is not to say I don't need help with a few pats on the back to release a particle of food now and again.

All of my problems are challenging, but pale into insignificance when I lose a friend to cancer, like Dr Jill White, for example – a consultant anaesthetist at NGH. She was a very popular lady who I had known for a number of years, since the time she was a registrar in the Gastric Clinic at NGH. Jill, even when she was very ill, wanted to know how I was and even towards the end of her life came to see me, in our self-build, with her husband Dick. I knew then that her light was fading, which made me very sad. I did admire her for her fighting spirit and love of life. Thoughts of her put the contents of this chapter in perspective.

AN ANXIOUS TURN OF EVENTS

I had been waiting for some scan results because of painful sinuses and my swallowing problem was gradually getting worse. I had told Mr Harrop that occasionally when I choked, Michael or friends had used the Heineken manoeuvre on me – instead of the proper name Heimlich – as certain words are harder for me to project and this is one of them. Mr Harrop got the joke straightaway and said that he would like some too, but Mr Gurr – who is the Ear Nose and Throat consultant (ENT) I had to see about my nose and throat and didn't know me – was not so switched on to my off-the-wall sense of humour and I had to explain!

The scans showed that I had a twisted septum which had properly been there for years and that my swallowing could be improved by stretching my oesophagus. I had also been complaining about a tooth which was causing me discomfort and I felt that it was also getting more painful. After an X-ray and photographs were taken, it was decided that it should be extracted. The problem was a calcium build-up caused by the Dry Mouth Syndrome – again as a result of surgery. I asked if I could have the tooth taken out at the same time as the other two procedures, as a kind of package deal! This was all agreed, but two days before the operation, a second lot of photographs and X-ray were ordered by Mr Harrop. As they worked on these, the mood of Sue, the nurse, and Rob, the technician in Maxillofacial, became more serious. They did not laugh when I said that Michael wanted to know if I could have a zip sewn into my neck, is case I needed my oesophagus stretched again – which I was told was certainly possible.

On the day of surgery, I was told by Mr Gurr that he would not be operating on my nose after all. Although they would still be taking my tooth out, a biopsy would be taken under anaesthetic, as Mr Harrop, having seen the X-rays and photographs, wasn't happy about the inflammation on the roof of my mouth. When Mr Gurr told me and showed me the photograph, I said, "Why? You're not looking for cancer, are you?" I remember saying that in an off-the-cuff sort of way, because I was cross that my nose was not going to be sorted. I was really looking forward to breathing more freely and not having to rely on a spray after so many years. He was very serious and had what I would interpret as a compassionate look on his face as he spoke. I just thought *What a nice man*. Clearly I did not want to hear any more, as I was psyched up for a general aesthetic and just wanted it all over and done with. I had already convinced myself that the inflammation would be Lichen Planus, as it had been identified at the time of the biopsy previously. I was so frustrated that they were not going to do my nose that I felt more like sulking and rang Michael to moan to.

The surgery stockings caused me more problems. Just like the last time eight years ago, when at 7am on the morning of the operation, my sister Sarah was helping me to pull them on. We both could not stop laughing. They were so tight. Maybe that's the whole point – releasing happy endorphins just before major surgery can't be bad!

The day after this relatively minor surgery, I was given the paperwork summarising the operation, which I didn't read straightaway. Why would I want to? I knew all I needed to know.

In order to stay positive, I had blocked out any thoughts that the biopsy might confirm the return of a malignant tumour. The ENT doctor came to see me and routinely discharged me with a follow-up appointment with Mr Harrop the following week. It wasn't until he'd gone that I spotted on the paperwork "SUSPECTED TUMOUR OF THE PALATE". It was a shock. I had to ask the nurse if that was correct. She was surprised the doctor hadn't told me. Of course he had. I just hadn't wanted to hear him.

Several weeks before all this started, I'd had a nightmare and had woken myself up screaming – something I had never done before. A few days later, I had another dream, screaming in my sleep at I don't know what. I was very frightened, but at the same time was very aware of many hands holding mine as if to comfort me. Naturally, I wondered why I was suddenly having dreams like this. I was about to find out. Knowing I had survived the terror of these dreams and remembering the reassurance of all those caring hands sustained me over the following weeks as the deterioration in my health unfolded. Although I was unaware that I needed it at the time, I have always believed that loved ones who have left this planet, will, if you ask them for help, be there for you by guiding and supporting you subconsciously. I know that some people think to believe in such things is nonsense, but it sits well with me.

The next week was awful for me, my family and close friends. We all knew I was having relatively straightforward surgery, but none of us suspected the cancer result, or if they did, no one dared mention it. On the day of my follow-up appointment with Mr Harrop and Anne Hicks, Michael came with me. I sensed a different atmosphere from the usual banter. We had known them and their staff for eight years and the usual friendly style always helped to make the visits easier. On this day though, we had a polite and pleasant preamble and no one mentioned the "elephant in the room".

I surprised myself when I walked in and, before I'd even sat down, I said, "Well, yes or no?" I had actually rehearsed this conversation with myself many times in the preceding week. Mr Harrop's face told me the answer before he even spoke. He was very sorry to have to tell me that it was a new Squamous Cell Carcinoma. "Pardon?" I said, as Mike mumbled under his breath. Wrong Answer. Mr H had to repeat the dreaded news. I do feel for the consultants and Ann Hicks as they care so much for their patients.

HERE WE GO AGAIN

The clinic was closing for lunch as Michael and I left. We walked down the corridor as the Maxillofacial nurses were coming the other way. Each one in turn gave us both hugs. Their support, as always, is fantastic. Over the eight and a half years, we have all got to know each other; their warmth and generosity of spirit has sustained us and meant so much when you are not sure what the future holds, especially when it is a 'repeat performance'.

In the two and a half weeks between diagnosis and the operation, I received so many wonderful cards, texts and telephone calls – all willing me to be strong and reminding me how much my family and friends mean to me, especially dear friends who have not had it easy themselves. Yvonne was already planning her work diary to make sure she was going to be free to take me to appointments and support Michael while I was in hospital.

In my more positive moments, I remembered how my cousin's husband, Simon Davies, coped when he was diagnosed with mouth cancer for the second time. His consultant told him: "Don't worry, Simon, we can cut the tumour out." Although his life changed considerably, he has managed to cope and adapt pretty well to his situation, with the help and support of his wife, my cousin, Pat, and his three daughters. Simon very generously bought ten copies of *TRILOGY* for the London hospital he was attending.

I remembered from the first time that as the drama unfolds, it can be as if it is happening to someone else. At times, I felt quite detached and lacking in emotion. The diagnosis was an unexpected twist that came bang in the midst of writing this [second] book. We had already planned how and where we would launch it in the following March, and organised and chosen the contributors. The publishers had begun work on the cover and Professor Nick Stafford and Nigella Lawson had agreed to offer their support. So, I had plenty to be thinking about, and if anyone thought I was a going to miss out on all the excitement just because a new cancer had come back, then they didn't know me very well.

A year previously, when Carol had her kidney removed, I remembered being so worried about her that I couldn't believe I was putting her through similar agony.

The day after receiving the diagnosis from Mr Harrop, we went to a party to celebrate Yvonne and Shane's daughter Kim's engagement to Paul. As far as I knew, no-one knew my situation, which was great. I intended to let my hair down and have a really good time, especially being there with Michael, Mark, Erika and her daughter Lisa, plus seeing many of the happy couple's friends and family – most of whom we knew.

It was a barn dance and, because of my back, I don't usually join in because they are fast and furious and involve lots of jumping about. As this time I was on painkillers and had had some bubbly, I hardly left the dance floor. I felt tremendous and absolutely loved it, feeling a huge warmth towards everyone. It was then I understood the saying "medication entertains the body whilst it heals" – my endorphins were certainly boosted. I loved watching Mark and Sam, Yvonne and Shane's son, barn dancing; something I thought I would never see. Apparently Yvonne and I were good entertainment, too! How could I possibly dwell on what was ahead of me surrounded by all this wonderful energy? It was a great party; a lovely atmosphere. Congratulations to Kim and Paul.

One of my first visitors during those two weeks was my friend Jenny Palmer-Jeffery. She knew the first time, long before anyone else including me that something really wasn't right, even though I just thought I had a cold and had been burning the candle at both ends. This time there were no clues – in fact, everyone kept telling me how well I looked – except for the fact I was complaining about my tooth. Jenny has always supported Facefax and the DB, and has always been a great ambassador within her well-connected circle of friends. The previous year, Jenny had been very ill herself and her life had been in the balance, so we were able to talk about how everything pales into insignificance when your life could be taken away. Being the positive fighter she is, her health is now back on track and she is socialising and travelling more than ever before – a wonderful example for us all.

One morning, Mark asked me, "Still feeling positive, Mum?" For me, there really was no choice. Many years ago, I was in a dark place. It was Reiki and hypnotherapy that turned my life around, along with diagnosis of some long-term allergies and my back being operated on. So, it is not that it has been easy. I just can't face that awful depression and dependency. After all, it is an attitude of mind and I am the only one who can change it.

There were two difficult days during the wait, when the contents of the post dropping on the doormat had a profound effect on my mood. First, came an appeal letter from the Samaritans, which gave me a jolt. It reminded me there were a lot of isolated and desperate people a lot worse off than me. Then, a letter from my insurance company telling me they wouldn't renew my life cover because of my second bout of cancer. Along with this, there was a card with three glamorous ladies in 1960s dresses on the front with the caption, "Friendship is always in fashion." What else could I do? I tore up the insurance letter and put up the card, because that is what is going to sustain me where I am in my life now.

I was worrying about the prospect of a dropped shoulder I had been told to expect, because Mr Harrop would be removing my neck muscle and nerve. How were my clothes going to hang? I asked Carol to get me a pair of "Dallas style" shoulder pads. As she too has had this problem, I suggested we both had one each so, together, we looked more balanced!

Sex, drugs and rock and roll. I have a lot to live up to. There always seems to be a negative side relating to the cause of mouth cancer – even Michael Douglas, the actor, had his take on it – but what about the lead that was used in newspaper print years ago? When I worked in advertising, I used to sneeze my head off when the first print run landed on our desks. As many people did, I used to lick my finger in order to turn the page – obviously not too clever for anyone intolerant to lead! But in those days, we knew no better. Who knows why it happens. It can be any number of reasons.

The day before the operation, I had until 4pm, which is when I was due at the Head and Neck Ward at Northampton General Hospital (NGH), to prepare for the operation the following day. I had booked myself some TLC; first with Tracey Bridger to restyle my hair and then with Michelle Dupry Sherratt to tint my eyebrows and eyelashes. Tracey is very artistic, both as a hairdresser and a photographer. She kindly took all the photographs at the Maharaja PR evening and made no charge. I knew these appointments would be a good idea because I was very nervous and emotional. It was good to be with friends who cared and knew me well enough to understand my frame of mind. I wanted to look so good that the medics would think twice before they cut into my neck and my face, if they had to – nonsense I know, but it was a good distraction and a morale booster too.

An hour before Yvonne was due to arrive and take me to NGH, I reread all the cards and texts I had received. I was aware that Sandy Reagan was sending me transference healing and Christine Gould had set up a group from Reiki Academy to send absent healing, for which I was very grateful and humbled. I am open to all kinds of positive energy and thoughts; I believe in the power they have and have done since I was a child.

As you can imagine, I didn't sleep the night before the operation, but was feeling quite calm when at 7am Michael and Yvonne arrived to escort me on my trolley to the door of the operating theatre.

The next thing I can remember was being wheeled back to the ward after quite some time in recovery. Just as we reached the entrance to the ward, we hit a slight bump which started me being sick. I remember feeling dreadful as I was wheeled past the staff and the nurses. Days later, I was told that they had taken one look at me and said that they did not expect me to be in hospital very long — that was nice to hear, but what made them think that when I felt so awful?

Day 3 – I was very much aware of my 'hamster face' with all its swelling and bruising. My experience last time told me that I should not worry and it would go down. Most importantly, I should not look in a mirror.

In my opinion, the staff and nurses on the Head and Neck Ward are just brilliant and work under very difficult circumstances. The patients they care for have so much going on. In my case, my blood pressure was an issue and my diet of course. Initially, because of my allergies and intolerance to dairy, gluten and soya, I was on Elemental 028, which contains all the vitamins, minerals and calories required to support me, and Maxijul, a carbohydrate powder that is sprinkled on food.

The drains in my neck were becoming very sore and uncomfortable when I lay down. I figured this was probably a sign of healing, so that was good. Anne Hicks popped in to see me and told me "the word on the street was that I was doing very well". I liked that; it made me smile. Ouch!

That night, I could not settle and like last time, eight years before, I paced the corridors like a caged lion. I even asked the nurses if they had any jobs for me to do. I assured them I did not want paying. They just smiled. Lying and sitting are not good for my back or my morale, and my blood pressure was an issue because of the pain, so I needed to generate some positive, happy endorphins rather than being a moaning Minnie. Then, a light bulb came on in my head. I need to go home!

Day 4 – At 5.30am I drank my nutritional drink, took my medicines and then had the luxury of having the bathroom to myself without feeling, if I took too long, I was hogging it as is my want. Not that I could do much with the drains in my neck – certainly no shower or much-needed hair wash. Returning to the ward, I tidied up my little area and wrote a paragraph for this book.

When Mr Harrop and his team arrived to do their rounds, I almost begged him to let me go home on the basis that I could be better in charge of my diet, which in turn would speed up my body's healing. The drains in my neck were discussed and as usual there was a bit of banter, which I love. Mr Harrop reminded me that I had just had major surgery and although I was doing well, it was only four days since the operation. I must admit that I did stamp my foot at one point with pure frustration, and after negotiations concerning blood pressure and nutrition and addressing the removal of the drains, it was agreed that if all continued to improve I could expect to be released "in two days". Brilliant! The next blood pressure reading taken was well down.

Having had quite a few operations in my lifetime – the first at age seven – my experiences have shown that consultants these days no longer see themselves as "God" and are nowhere near as remote and offhand as they used to be when talking to their patients. It makes such a difference to a person who may be feeling vulnerable, propped up in bed and surrounded by medics, and with very little control over their own destiny. I have a great respect for anyone who has studied so long and so hard, and in my case, I am extremely grateful that they did. I must also add that NHS staff have always treated me well.

Within the hour, I had one drain removed, which I confess I wasn't looking forward to as last time it had been a painful experience, but it was another sign of progress. If it went well, the other one would be removed soon afterwards. Thanks to the skill of the nurse and, much to my relief, it came out quite easily. I could feel my optimism lifting and my humour being buoyed. When Mr Gurr the ENT consultant did his rounds he would look over at me and graciously nod. I nodded and smiled back. It was all very amusing. Mr Tarwin, a very jovial character who had taken my tooth out, also made me laugh as he passed by. At teatime, the second drain came out – freedom. I knew I could look forward to that shower and hair wash very soon now.

That evening, my sister, Sarah, came up from Dorset and we had a good catch up. I am not saying my speech was perfect, but eight years of practising voice projection stood me in good stead. With the prosthesis in place and having had my oesophagus stretched, which seemed to help, I felt that although I used a lot of energy, my communication was pretty effective.

The following day was Saturday and Mr Harrop's registrar, Mr Parbhoo, was on duty. He seemed pleased with my progress, but was still cautious about pronouncing if I could go home the next day. A decision would be made in the morning. I was feeling very optimistic and asked him when I would be able to drive, bearing in mind how painful my neck and shoulder were. As I write this, eight weeks on, they still can be. For that reason, Mr Parbhoo advised in about three months. I then said my next goal was to visit my friend, Trudie, in South Africa. When did he think this could be? I don't think he told me, but instead asked me where in South Africa? It turned out he had lived there with his uncle and had worked at the Children's Red Cross Hospital in Cape Town. I told him about Trudie's guesthouse in Stellenbosch, near Cape Town, and the fact that she now lived near the Kruger Park in a town called Hoedspruit. To my surprise, he knew it. And so to my next question, about taking Malaria tablets, which always usually upset me. He suggested spraying my body and clothes with DEET malaria sprays. I was delighted to have a solution to this problem, which had concerned me for some time. I really did not want to go down with Malaria. So thank you, Mr Parbhoo. You made my day – two important questions answered.

That afternoon, my cousin, Vicky, came with Michael and my sister at visiting time. It was lovely to see them all. Michael had collected Vicky from the station. She had travelled down from Manchester, where she had been at a Robbie Williams concert the night before. Vicky told me Robbie had sung "Angels" and suggested to the audience they dedicate it to someone they had lost, or knew had been through a difficult time. She had dedicated it to me. I love her dearly and now you can understand why.

In the evening, when Michael returned after taking Vicky back to the station, so she could return home to Burley-in-Wharfdale near Leeds, he brought Sarah and Mark with him. It was very emotional for me to see Mark, who had returned from a holiday in Bulgaria – booked months before we knew I needed treatment. I was very pleased he hadn't been around during the operation and in the early days of recovery. Then, to top everything, Michael produced an iPad which he'd known I had wanted for some time, and said, "That is for being a brave girl." Mark then exclaimed, "Oh no! iPad lessons! It was bad enough with the laptop!" My powers of concentration over the next few weeks were a bit up-and-down, so he didn't need to worry for a while.

A special thank you to Yvonne for keeping my family and friends, including Trudie in South Africa, informed of my progress during that week. I hear, Yvonne, that you did a sterling job. I am pleased that this part of the story had a happy ending.

Great news! Mr Parbhoo agreed I could go home. I always say, never outstay one's welcome and leave on a high… and that is just how I feel.

HOME SWEET HOME

Sarah waited for me to return home before she left for Dorset. Her younger daughter was pregnant with her first child and so it was important for Sarah to be back home as the due date was approaching.

Suddenly, I felt very vulnerable. No nurse offering painkillers. I had been warned that the pain in my neck and chest would get worse before it got better. The first night was awful, up and down the whole time. Then, there were the scars around my neck to tend to. *Nurse, where are you when I need you?* But I didn't, for a moment, regret coming home. My reward for getting through the night was two delicious cups of coffee, first thing, which Michael always brings me. They have to cool down a bit before drinking though, so the heat does not distort my obturator which was made of a plastic-based material. To make it ill-fitting would damage my mouth.

The first day at home on my own was a new challenge. The aforementioned pain was really beginning to take hold and the paracetamol and ibuprofen I was taking just wasn't keeping it under control. For the first time since the days before the operation I resorted to taking Tramadol and then all I wanted to do was sleep. The next day, Michael asked me if I would like him to take the week off. YES PLEASE!

Kay Hughes called in and taught me how to use reflexology pressure points on my hands to help with the feeling of sickness due to the painkillers and I suspect lack of food, which I was not particularly interested in.

Frankie Button kindly helped me with my neck, where the drains had been removed; the stitches made it look like I had a small porcupine sitting on my shoulder. They were so sharp! Was this an example of "man stitching"? A question I was certainly going to put to Mr Harrop at our next meeting. Whatever, they certainly weren't going to come undone! Frankie also helped me wash my hair, which was just bliss! As always, she had brought me some delicious homemade soups and an elderberry sorbet with fruits picked from her garden. Next, a lovely surprise, a fabulous mixed plant arrangement arrived via Interflora from my relatives in Yorkshire.

I was clearly starting to relax and so forgot to concentrate on drinking, at which point, the liquid food and drink came back down my nose – not a pleasant experience or a good look. I was not ready to party just yet!

On my fifth day at home, I attended my first post-operative appointment with Mr Harrop. He was happy with my mouth and confirmed that continuing to use Chlorhexidine mouthwash three times a day was aiding the healing. In addition, I was using Arnica Gel, which I swear by, on my neck, shoulder and chest – a brilliant aid to natural healing.

Mr Harrop then addressed my neck and agreed his work looked pretty brutal, but apparently the stitching had been done by him (oh no!) and was a recommended new technique which promised much neater scarring. Well, I had no choice but to trust his word. Michael said he thought I looked like a chipmunk because of the swollen right cheek, and the stitches and scar looked like I was a pyjama case with a zip! He usually sits to my right when we have an early morning coffee and all the procedures were on my right side. It caused him great amusement. Thank goodness I could see the funny side too, even at this time of heightened anxiety, waiting to hear if I would need radiotherapy. I was keeping my fingers crossed for a lucky escape from this, as I had been granted last time.

A long week passed. Then, I had a call from Anne Hicks to say I would NOT be needing radiotherapy. The feeling of relief was immense as I feared any further invasive treatment would finish me off. I had lost three quarters of a stone in weight, which was not good as I had not put all the weight on that I had lost eight years ago and was feeling very weak indeed. This good news was just the boost I needed.

By the end of the following week, the pain of the obturator was becoming increasingly difficult to bear and meant I had to increase the painkillers. On the Monday morning, I rang Maxillofacial who saw me straightaway and booked me into theatre the following day. It turned out that the healing and reducing of the swelling had resulted in the obturator no longer fitting correctly inside my mouth.

As advised by Anne Hicks, Maxillofacial Clinical Nurse Specialist at NGH:

Your first operation was: Excision Squamous Cell Carcinoma from right lateral tongue and reconstruction with a radial Forearm Free flap. Surgery also included a Tracheostomy and a selective neck dissection and fitting of Percutaneous Endoscopic Gastrostomy (PEG). This information is in *TRILOGY,* the original book.

Your second operation was: for a new cancer in your Right Maxilla (upper jaw). This is not a recurrence of your original cancer, it was a Partial Maxillectomy and fitting of obturator plus a radical neck dissection. Feeding was through a naso-gastric tube until oral intake was possible.

The third operation was: Removal of obturator, re-modelling of bung and cleaning of cavity. This happened because of the pain you were in.

The histological examination confirmed that the cancer was completely removed, with clear margins. The neck nodes were negative and therefore no radiotherapy was recommended. A regime of monthly clinical follow-up appointments will be started with Mr Harrop and me (Anne Hicks). You will also have regular appointments with the Prosthodontist (Pamela Hall) to ensure the obturator is comfortable and to support your management.

WHEN THE GOING GETS TOUGH, THE TOUGH GET GOING

I must admit I felt very sorry for myself returning for yet another general anesthetic so soon, but I also knew that things didn't feel right.

As it was day surgery this time – and I had experienced this before when I had the biopsy done and the tooth removed – you walk escorted to the theatre from the day ward. The first time it amused me walking down the corridor with the staff standing outside the numbered theatres waiting for their patients. In fact, I remembered smiling at them and thinking this was not a good look, walking past all these people dressed in an oversized gown and theatre slippers. My escort this time was a lovely gentleman, a fatherly figure, who made me feel cared for. This meant a lot; walking down the corridor to whichever number theatre had been allocated to me, I felt like a lamb on its way to slaughter and vulnerable – probably because it was so soon after my big operation. Nobody got a smile!

As I said before, after the bigger op, my thoughts while lying in the recovery area were a mixture of a) feeling awful b) trying to work out what a prosthesis in one's mouth actually feels like c) whether I would actually ever be able to talk again and d) being sick with quite a lot of blood around my mouth, which was feeling extremely dry.

I was given wet paper hankies to clean my mouth and only tiny sips of water, just enough to moisten my mouth while I waited for my blood pressure to go down. For me, that is additionally frustrating, because I am never aware that it is up. When the nurse sat beside me writing up her notes, she checked my age and told me that I was doing very well and thanks be to God – a lovely thing to say. This was said to me on both occasions by different staff. It was good to be reminded that I should be thankful, but at that moment, God was right at the bottom of my list. But as I lay there, I imagined the potential for a medical sitcom with so much going on around me with other patients and medics. Even then, I had not lost my sense of humour. Life is never boring, not even in recovery.

Later that day when I was discharged, my mouth and the obturator were more comfortable. I had gone without painkillers all day and was using hypno healing tools on myself that I had used on others when in practice. It had to be the way forward. In other words, rather than concentrating on the pain and using heavy painkillers, I was using the distraction techniques which I referred to many times in *TRILOGY.* I am talking about mild pain as opposed to deep pain, now. I am sure deep pain can be managed by distraction, but I can't honestly say I have managed it myself without the help of some painkillers. Fellow patients of mouth cancer will know this is a difficult journey and fighting it is not easy.

For some reason, I struggled with the next two days, even though my mouth felt a lot more comfortable. Maybe it was the aftermath of more anesthetic and medication in my system. Yvonne rang and must have sensed my low mood, because she asked if she could call in and say hi. I agreed; it was a good decision, because as a good friend and a trained counsellor, she encouraged me to express my feelings. We also discussed my diet as I had realised the only way forward was to puree everything to a very fine consistency, and to think about meals in this way was just too much for me to handle in these early days. I am so grateful to Yvonne, Joy, Frankie, Manjeet and Erika for helping me with the tasty meals they prepared for me to freeze. As I write this piece, I am eight weeks on from the second operation and I am only just beginning to use my imagination to be creative with tasty meals myself. I know that Kay Owen, the dietician, and Anne Hicks are emphatic that correct nutrition plays such a critical part in the body's recovery and that was now very important to me.

The following day, my spirits were still a bit low. Then, I happened across, quite by chance, an interview with Christopher Reeve's son on TV. He lost his father in such tragic circumstances when he was only fifty-two, having dealt with the aftermath of such a devastating accident – so how dare I be miserable? This somehow brought me to my senses.

Looking back now, I am quite sure all the medication and anesthetics were suppressing my drive and will to survive, because for no apparent reason, those two days were exceptionally and surprisingly hard for me.

MOVING ON

Thank goodness it didn't last. I woke up the next day to a beautiful sunny Saturday, which began with coffee on the patio at 6.30am. In fact, I spent much of the day outside snatching as much vitamin D as I could. I texted friends to say that I was feeling stronger and invited them to visit as they had requested me to. I felt driven to send this email to Anne Hicks:

"I have turned a corner and had my first glass of fizz on Saturday evening with Manjeet and Sushel which tasted like nectar."

On Sunday, I woke up with the same attitude, so I plucked up the courage to go out with wonky lips and clothes not hanging right due to my right shoulder and weight loss. As Mike would say 'Get a grip.' His army background often comes to the fore when he thinks one should toughen up! He took me to a charity event for the DB organised by Christine, so I could see the volunteers and thank them all for their support. I joked that I didn't like to miss anything and want to be kept in the loop. They are all doing a wonderful job.

The book was also on my mind. I was only halfway through all the things I had to do and time was pressing on. Vicky Smith had very kindly offered to type up my notes, because with a dropped shoulder and post-neck surgery, sitting for any length of time at my laptop was painful. Short spells were okay to write an email, but the intensity of concentrating for longer periods was no good at all. So, I wrote the rest of my script in longhand on my lap, collating notes that I had written when things came into my mind. These were written in hospital, at home in the middle of the night or early hours of the morning, in fact, anytime I felt driven to capture my thoughts. It was also important to keep in touch with the contributors, as Carol was also doing. It was important to assure them we were still going ahead with the book.

So, Vicky and I sorted out some dates and a huge sense of relief descended upon me.

The glorious summer weather continued – perfect for convalescing, writing and friend's visits, which all helped me to keep going forward and meet the health challenges head on.

After losing so much weight, the way my clothes fitted me became an issue. Michael suggested we went to a children's store, but as he won't go to the "Big Man's Shop", I couldn't see why I should! Unfortunately, Gary Osbourne at Ossie's had sold out of small sizes as it was now sale time, but it was just nice to speak to him and Jamie, who helps in the shop, and catch up.

Lovely cards and presents kept arriving. Flowers from Trudie in South Africa, followed by six bottles of sparkling wine, which had been specially chosen so that it was not too dry and very light. Apart from the odd occasion, when I forgot to concentrate and it came back down my nose, this was very welcome and kept my spirits lifted. Thank you so much for all the energy and kindness you all showered upon me when I needed it most.

It has been said to me several times: "It just isn't fair this has happened to you again, Ann." All I can say to that is, of course nobody wants to be ill, but without these challenges we would not experience such wonderful acts of kindnesses. Under perfect circumstances, we would all be very selfish and self-absorbed. I think to see people pull together in times of need – whatever that need may be – is wonderful and an inspiration to witness. It makes everyone take stock of their lives and evaluate whether to be a participator or an onlooker, to the extreme. One Sunday evening, Michael was having a moan about the news on TV. Then, we went on to watch *The White Queen* on BBC. It was set in the period leading up to Richard III being crowned. I turned to Mike and said, "You think we have problems! At least we are not going round cutting each other's heads off and slitting throats" and I laughed. Michael very quickly retorted, "Try mouth cancer."

I was increasingly aware that my shoulder seemed to be seizing up. As Carol had experienced a similar problem, I knew I should telephone Anne Hicks to ask her about physiotherapy. Because an appointment with NGH would take a number of weeks, Anne asked me if I knew anyone who could help, as leaving it that long might result in a frozen shoulder. A chilling thought! I contacted

Bill MacKay, who I hadn't seen for ten years. He had treated me after my back surgery and we'd got on very well. Fortunately, he was still practising and was able to see me the next day. My shoulder felt so much easier, even after one session with him. I knew that I would be given a programme of exercises which at times would be painful. Arnica (which Bill approves of) and two paracetamol nightly seemed to keep this under control. As I write this, it is eight weeks since the operation and four weeks into the physio. Although I don't want to finish up looking like 'Mrs Universe' on my right side, I am really pleased to report that my shoulders now look more equalised. Bill knows that I have another two and a half months to go until I need to wear a special outfit to a ball. I have every confidence in his skill. I am using a lot of visualisation to see myself as I want to be. I have used this technique in the past with my hypnotherapy clients, but I do have plenty of work to do!

Comment from Bill Mackay MSc MCSP, Witty Pask & Buckingham, 56 Billing Road, Northampton NN1 5DB Tel: 01604 601641

Generally speaking, as an out-patient physiotherapy practice, we do not receive many referrals following major cancer surgery to the head, neck and throat, but in the past, I have had experience of patients who have had trauma to one or more of those areas.

I first met Ann when she was under my care following a major back operation in 2003. At that time, I was impressed with her well-developed sense of humour coupled with a single-minded dedication to getting back to full fitness as quickly as possible. Two years later, she then had the misfortune to contract cancer of the mouth and tongue, which was treated surgically. I only knew of this after I bumped into her in a local supermarket a year or so after her tongue and mouth surgery. She made light of it and it was clear that Ann's approach to surmounting this new problem was the same as the one that she had adopted to her spinal trauma.

In July 2013, I was reacquainted with Ann following a recurrence of her mouth cancer, which was operated on some three weeks earlier. This time the surgery was more radical and Ann had had to undergo removal of lymph gland and nerves, resulting in a variety of musculoskeletal problems involving her neck, shoulder girdle and shoulder joint. These, of course, were in addition to the obvious ones involving her soft palate and having to wear an intrusive prosthesis, which would need many months to accommodate to her mouth. A thorough post-operative assessment is important to enable the physiotherapist to establish what the musculoskeletal problems are, in order to prioritise treatment options. In Ann's case, it was important to prevent a frozen shoulder from developing, and to strengthen the residual muscles in the neck and shoulder girdle to compensate for lost muscle tissue, which meant working on compensatory techniques to strengthen her shoulder elevators and shoulder blade retractors. Additionally, postural modifications and re-education was needed. Her neck stiffness needed to be addressed by manual fibrous release techniques in conjunction with passive, assisted active and active mobilisation exercises. We then progressed to strengthening exercises, initially in a static position and then dynamically, gradually increasing the strength throughout full range.

As ever, Ann directed one hundred per cent effort into maximising her recovery. I must note here that in her positive, upbeat approach, in conjunction with her diligence and sense of humour, she reminded me of the same spirit and resilience shown by the numerous patients I had encountered during my time serving in the RAF when working at the Defence Services Medical Rehabilitation Centre at Headley Court.

As far as eating is concerned, it is all a bit messy and I could not envisage eating out in a restaurant. Then, there is the issue of asking them to blend the meal. Anyway, I managed it on Ella Bennett, my sister-in-law's birthday. I thought if she could do it – she has MS and has to be helped – then so could I. The Indian restaurant where the party was held kindly blended my Malay curry. Since then, the Maharaja has blended a T/A for me once a week, so I now feel more confident in asking other restaurants to do the same. Kissing everyone goodbye at the end of the evening was an unexpected challenge, as I can't form a kiss anymore. I don't know if this will be forever, but it did hit me quite hard when I realised. There are others far worse off than me. It is a case of adjustment – something mouth, head and neck cancer patients have to get used to. When your condition is so obvious, there is nowhere to hide. When I have listened to clients seeking help at the DB, whatever type of cancer they have had or have, they are often very emotional, but the fact they are facing up to it and seeking help is positive and a good sign.

Neither Carol nor myself are 'shrinking violets' and I am sure we would quickly become depressed about the challenges of having had mouth cancer if we couldn't be out and about, regularly socialising. We owe it to our friends and family who help pull us through, regardless of how we eat, drink, speak or look.

My first appointment with Pam Hall, the prosthodontist, was looming and I was apprehensive as the obturator felt loose again, though not painful this time. Carol came with me and witnessed me clutching Maxillofacial dental nurse Anna's hand as Pam removed the prosthesis from my mouth, for the first time with no anesthetic. Just the thought of it being removed had made me very tense. The area was cleaned and checked. It all felt very strange. Mr Harrop was there too and so was Rob the technician. Having gone through this, I knew I would feel a lot more relaxed the next time when they would be taking an impression to adjust the obturator. This would take about two hours, during which time – without it – I would be unable to speak. When the time came, I did try, but I was barely audible – the energy to project my voice was too great to overcome. Luckily, I had gone prepared with Carol by my side and a pen and paper. I asked Pam if that then would be the end of it. "No," she said, "you have a long way to go yet." Twelve months at least, which totally threw me. I don't have an abundance of patience at the best of times – I know, because this has been well and truly tested many times in my life.

I had to learn how to take the obturator out and put it back in again for myself. For hygiene purposes, I need to do this twice a day, for no more than ten minutes each time. The very thought of this responsibility petrified me, but I knew I had no choice if I wanted to continue to make good progress and avoid further complications. Even so, how on earth was I ever going to get used to having this foreign object in my mouth?

As the swelling receded, my bottom lip, which was lopsided, didn't look quite so out of line and my neck scars were beginning to fade. Clearly the Bio-Oil I was using to heal the scars was having an effect and Mr Harrop was right about the new stitching technique. Sorry, Mr Harrop, for being so sniffy about your needlework. I missed out on one day of using Bio-Oil on my scars. The result was soreness and tightness, so I knew the oil helped a lot. The same applies to physio. I only missed one day and everything felt like it was seizing up. Of course, these were early days and one might say all this was normal and I accepted that, but my experiences have encouraged me to be consistent and to do EVERYTHING each day. Otherwise, I knew there would be a penalty to pay and I would feel worse.

It became obvious that as the healing process continued and the swelling reduced, my jaw wasn't opening very easily. How had that happened? I was talking quite a bit, with lots of jaw exercises. Michael couldn't understand it; he would have loved a bit of peace and quiet. Consequently, I was finding it more and more difficult to eat. I can't chew but I do need to be able to open my mouth wide enough to use a spoon and fork, so once again I called Anne Hicks who suggested getting a 'Therabite' through my GP. A Therabite is a contraption, a bit like a car jack, designed to prise open the jaws. Its official description is a 'jaw motion rehabilitation system'.

What a coincidence. Approximately three years ago, Facefax charity gave funds to the Maxillofacial Clinic to buy six Therabites for use by patients who were unable to open their jaws after surgery. Little did I know then that I would need one myself. I remember thinking at the time how awful it must be for people in that position, and as a Trustee of Facefax, I didn't hesitate in agreeing to give the money. They can now be obtained on prescription through a GP.

At my next appointment with Pam to check the obturator, I showed her and Paul the technician the Therabite, which looked just so big for my mouth. They both reassured me it would have the desired effect eventually. I had no choice if I didn't want my jaw to get worse. I'd thought, eight years ago, this mouth cancer business was high maintenance. I knew nothing then!

In the midst of all this, Trudie and Yvonne kept asking me when we were going for a holiday to South Africa. We had all talked about going to Trudie's to celebrate Michael's seventieth birthday in November (2013). Mark, very generously, offered to pay his father's airfare as a birthday present. What a great place for me to recuperate. I texted Anne Hicks to ask if she thought I would be ready to travel in November. She agreed it would do us both the world of good. She knew we would be as well looked after as we had been under similar circumstances eight years previously. I googled Cape Town and Johannesburg Hospitals and found both had a Maxillofacial Clinic and specialist surgeons. It had more to do with the obturator really as it would still need to be regularly checked and I needed the reassurance that if anything were to happen, experts would be close at hand. A kind of insurance you could say, just in case – not that I really expected to use it as my appointments at NGH Maxillofacial are very regular.

IMPROVEMENTS

As I mentioned earlier, for a while I had been using visualisation techniques, as I had done with clients when I had been a practising hypnotherapist. Seeing myself in my mind's eye as I would like to be was a critical part of my recovery, rather than looking in the mirror and seeing my lip and my shoulder as they really were.

At ten weeks, I realised that there were changes: my lip was getting straighter, the physio – though painful at times – was at least paying off and my shoulder was definitely getting higher as the muscles strengthened. No need for a shoulder pad, after all. I am reminded of the saying: no pain, no gain!

Wow! I also realised I had put on 2lbs, so I popped into Ossie's in desperation and Sally, Gary's daughter, found me two pairs of trousers – thank goodness! Julie Barnes-Ward bought me an outfit, too. Originally, she'd thought of getting something for me to relax in, like a onesie, but then she decided I would look like Andy Pandy and opted for a very nice jumper and scarf, which I love. I am really pleased you changed your mind… thank you, Julie.

Swallowing is still an issue if food gets stuck, but I am learning to be very careful as the heartburn it causes is awful. My cousin's wife, Lesley, inspired me on a recent visit – just like she did the first time – with some tasty recipes that would work blended. As soon as I have finished writing, I intend to become more imaginative when it comes to meal times. The obturator was settling in and I felt more at ease with it – well, only just! The real pressure was taking it out for ten minutes twice a day for hygiene purposes and not being able to talk very well if I had to. The knack of projecting, which I first learned eight years ago, has been a godsend. Even if I need to speak without the obturator in place, it does take a lot of energy and, I am not very audible, but I can manage.

A problem with my right ear has surfaced and it is being investigated and soon to be resolved, I hope. I am persevering with the Therabite and counting my blessings. I will not live in fear of cancer a third time. Carol and I are enjoying life and there is still so much left to do.

FINALLY

This is my cut-off point and although I have a long way still to go, I am reminded constantly that telling my story and writing this book would not have been possible without the help of:

My friends, who made my meals when my interest in food was so low. Those meals have sustained me and given me the energy to go forward.

Friends and family, who have kept my spirits up with all their visits, cards and presents.

Anne Hicks and the Maxillofacial staff, Mr Harrop and his team, who are all so caring and supportive.

Physiotherapist Bill MacKay, who puts me through it, but makes me laugh – sometimes there are tears running down my cheeks. Laughter is such great therapy.

Christine Gould and Friends of Reiki Academy.

A big thank you to Vicky for deciphering my notes and typing them up since the operation.

To Chris Owens for helping us with the technical side and putting the work on disc for the publisher to proofread and edit.

To Tony Boullemier, our editor for *TRILOGY*, advising us regarding choice of publisher and answering any questions we had. It was very good of him to help us, having only just finished his own second book called *The Little Book of Monarchs* – www.boullemierbooks.co.uk

And, of course, to Carol for all her support and bringing humour into a journey that we both know is challenging. We have proved there is NO TIME FOR CANCER. I know that Carol has also had help with the book and I will leave her to add her own thanks to this list.

Whilst the manuscript is with the publisher, we are going down to Eastbourne to see Tony and Sandra Grech and onto Hayling Island to see Yvonne and Ken Hare, dear friends who we have known for a very long time. Then, on to Dorset to visit my younger niece, Jessica, and her husband, Phil, to meet the newest addition to our family – their baby daughter Zara. We will celebrate as we did at the end of writing *TRILOGY*, which coincidently coincides with new life coming into the world. Congratulations to you both, Jessica and Phil, and to my sister, her first grandchild and Hana, Jessica's sister, a niece.

FUTURE

In June 2014, Sharon Wright, Dental Hygienist at the Maxillofacial Facial Unit, will be trekking the highest mountain in Africa, Kilimanjaro, to help raise money for the Facefax Association.

Emma Eccles will be joining Sharon in Africa and she will also be running in the London Marathon in April 2014.

If you would like to make a donation, please call the Dunstone Bennett Suite on 07541 998711 or contact the Maxillofacial reception on 01604 545598 or email: dunstonebennett@gmail.com

Chapter 4

MAXILLOFACIAL UNIT

ORAL CANCER: A SURGEON'S SUMMARY

Mr W P Smith FDSRCS FRCS (Ed) FRCS (Eng)
Consultant Maxillofacial Surgeon

In the 1970s, cancer of the head and neck, which included mouth, jaws, throat and voice box, was a disease characteristically of elderly gentlemen who smoked excessively and drank spirits. Since then, the pattern and presentation of head and neck cancers has changed particularly in the last ten years. Sadly, we are seeing an increasing number of patients with head and neck cancer, to such an extent that it is now almost considered an epidemic within medical circles.

The patients are also changing, becoming younger and just as likely to be a man as a woman – although many of them are smokers, but not invariably drinkers. Sadly, patients often present late, having failed to attend their doctor or their dentist at an early stage when it is recognised that early diagnosis is more likely to be cured than late disease.

Treatment for head and neck cancers has also changed over the last thirty years when radiotherapy was the first line of treatment often offered before surgery. The rationale for such treatment was that surgery in the 1970s and 1980s was frequently described as mutilating, because reconstruction of the defect that resulted from cancer removal was crude and resulted in a very poor quality of life. Moreover, the radiotherapy techniques in the 1970s and 1980s were unsophisticated, which resulted in extreme severe side effects that were relentless.

Modern surgery and modern radiotherapy techniques have nevertheless improved the quality of life and outcomes for patients with head and neck cancer. Surgery is now considered the first line of treatment for many patients particularly with cancer of the mouth and radiotherapy techniques are much more refined to ensure that the side effects are reduced and the quality of life improved. Patients with head and neck cancer now do have a better quality of life, but those with late disease continue to die on a regular basis mainly as a result of the extensive disease at presentation, rather than the improved techniques in treatment.

The future for head and neck cancer revolves around prevention rather than treatment and the cessation of smoking, reduction of alcohol consumption and the prevention of HPV 16 spread (a virus that causes cancer of the cervix in women, which is now implicated with cancer of the tonsil and root of the tongue) will be the goals for the medical profession and public alike in the medium to long term.

Mr Colin Harrop FDS RCPS FRCS (OMFS)
Consultant Oral and Maxillofacial Surgeon

Oral cancer has been increasing in incidence for some years and whilst it remains largely a disease of old age, we are seeing increasing numbers of younger patients, particularly men, with oral cancer. The majority of oral cancer in the UK (70%) is related to use of tobacco and alcohol. However, we are increasingly recognising the importance of human papilloma virus as a potential cause. This is a widespread virus, which in most people causes no significant difficulty. The immune system in some patients, however, seems to have difficulty dealing with the virus and these patients are at higher risk of developing oral cancer.

The increasing incidence makes it vitally important to publicise the harmful effects of smoking and drinking and to ensure that new oral cancers are diagnosed and treated quickly.

The prognosis for a patient with oral cancer is significantly improved if the cancer is small and if there has been no spread of the cancer to other areas such as lymph nodes in the neck.

Early diagnosis not only helps to ensure a better prognosis. It also allows aggressive treatments with less disfiguring surgery and less profound effects on speech, chewing and swallowing.

The main curative treatments for oral cancer are surgery and radiotherapy, although there is an increasing use of chemotherapy as an adjunct (especially with radiotherapy). It is often easier for patients to comprehend the concept of surgery and what the potential effects might be. These effects can be frightening for patients and often radiotherapy may be seen as a less challenging treatment. The side effects of radiotherapy, however, can also be unpleasant both in the early stages (sore skin, sore mouth, tiredness) and later (dry mouth, taste disturbance, damage to the bone of the jaws).

Modern management of oral cancer now involves discussion of every case by a multidisciplinary team to ensure that the patient is offered the most appropriate treatment. The team also includes dieticians, speech and language therapists, and clinical nurse specialists who are critical to the support of patients before, during and after treatment.

In addition to this support, many patients derive benefit from a number of alternative therapies. For some patients, these can help to cope with the many negative feelings that accompany cancer and its treatment. Many patients are at risk of significant anxiety and depression, which compound an already difficult period.

Prevention of oral cancer probably remains the most important aim and in addition to behaviour changes around smoking and alcohol, future developments may include vaccination against human papilloma virus which is already used in the prevention of cervical cancer. Good evidence of its benefit in the prevention of oral cancer, however, is not yet available.

MAXILLOFACIAL TECHNOLOGISTS

Maxillofacial technologists are a group of professionals that work within the hospital environment and share a passion for manufacturing bespoke medical devices or appliances. Their work is mainly of a maxillofacial nature, but because of their ability to manipulate materials, they are also involved with constructing many different types of medical appliances for other hospital specialisms and frequently work with ENT, Plastic Surgery or Dermatology Consultants and their colleagues.

As nearly all the medical devices manufactured by MTs are of the bespoke nature (i.e. made specifically for a particular patient), it is important that accuracy and attention to detail figures highly in the work ethic.

They need to work within tolerances of a thousandth of an inch to achieve results that are going to fit comfortably and securely without causing any further damage to skin, tissue, teeth or bone when being worn.

Maxillofacial Technologists start out life as Dental Technologists. This gives them a thorough grounding in material sciences, oral, head and neck anatomy, impression and moulding techniques, the treatment of oral and facial trauma, an understanding of the complexities of occlusion (how upper and lower teeth meet and work together) and many other dextrous skills in manipulating materials and operating specialist equipment. Dental Technologists train further to become maxillofacial technologists and work primarily in the hospital environment. When it comes to treating patients with oral cancer, this gives them direct access to other members of the team and more importantly gives them access to the patient.

Maxillofacial Technologists play a very important role in the treatment of patients with oral and/or facial cancer, being involved at the planning, surgical intervention and rehabilitation stages of their treatment. They work very closely with a team of professionals to aid the patient through what is a most difficult time and in some instances will continue to see them for the rest of their life.

So what does a Maxillofacial Technologist do within the team that specifically treats oral cancer and how can they affect patient care and treatment?

Oral cancer affects patients in different ways, presenting itself in the mouth in different forms and occuring in different areas of the oral cavity. There are many different types of cancer that can occur in the mouth and all have differing treatment regimen, making it necessary to identify what the tumour is. Some are slow to develop and some are aggressive, developing quickly and spreading rapidly. Where the Maxillofacial Technologist is concerned, cancer in the lower jaw has a different treatment pathway to cancers in the upper jaw.

The top priority when treating any oral cancer is the total removal of the tumour and this is carried out by the surgeons in theatre, followed by preparation of the patient for recovery. This may involve using reconstruction techniques with titanium plates, flaps, bone grafts or medical devices. Maxillofacial Technologists manufacture these medical devices, which can take the form of a healing plate, metal splinting or a device used in the upper jaw called an obturator – all of which are fabricated before any surgery takes place.

LOWER JAW

Cancer in the lower jaw requiring intervention can at worst lead to surgical reconstruction using titanium bars and plates – used to replace bone – and flaps or skin grafts used to replace tissue. A flap is a piece of tissue that is taken from another part of the patient's body and used to fill the hole left by the tumour that has been removed. Sometimes, flaps can be harvested that have bone attached, which can at the same time be used to reconstruct some of the lower jaw. However, following surgery and a period of healing, the mouth may feel and behave differently.

It is not unusual for patients to experience some of the following problems:

- limited opening – not being able to open the mouth as widely as before.
- restricted tongue movement.
- a lack of natural ridge.
- a dry mouth.
- temporary or, in some cases permanent, numbness.
- loss of many or all natural teeth.
- reduction in tongue size and function.
- other minor problems like control of saliva flow from the mouth.

Obviously, speech is going to be affected to some extent if surgery interferes or encroaches upon the tongue.

It takes a good while for the surgery to heal, for things to settle down and for the patient to become accustomed to their new mouth.

It is not until this stage that the Maxillofacial Technologist will become involved with restoring the mouth, hopefully, back to full function, enabling the patient to eat, speak and be understood, smile and look as normal as possible.

They do this by working very closely with the patient and a dental surgeon, fabricating bespoke lower dental prosthetics (a special denture) that fits the remaining teeth and tissues, replacing any lost bone height and any missing teeth.

This denture is crafted with great care, taking into account the new shape and structure of the mouth, the patient's needs and desires, their current state of health and with an eye on future health developments of the patient that may or may not occur. We expect this denture to aid patients to chew food, helping them to recover quicker by eating more enjoyably and making available a wider choice of food textures, sizes and consistencies to be consumed. This denture can also restore the facial height and 'pads' out the cheeks to restore facial balance and improve the patient's appearance. This in turn can re-establish confidence in going out to meet and greet people and enable life to carry on with the world being none the wiser. They can, in some instances, improve on speech by helping with the pronunciation of words. Stability and retention of the denture can sometimes be aided if necessary by using implants, but this is not always possible due to bone condition, positioning and the possibility of radiotherapy treatment – all of which can have a detrimental effect on the implant's ability to 'take' or join physically to the bone.

UPPER JAW

The upper jaw, or maxilla, has the further complication of being in very close proximity to the nasal cavity. The bone covering the palate is not very thick and surgery to this area can result in a hole between the mouth and the nose. This hole or opening needs to be blocked up and there are ways of achieving this surgically using a flap, or it can be carried out prosthetically using an obturator.

What is an Obturator?

The dictionary definition for 'Obturator' is:
> *An object, device or body part that closes or obstructs an opening or access to a cavity.*
> *An Obturator – from a Maxillofacial viewpoint – is a "dental plate" worn by the patient that blocks up a hole in the roof of their mouth (palate).*

Obturators for maxillofacial patients vary in their design and shape and can be manufactured using different materials including plastic (acrylic), metal and silicone. Most obturators also replace teeth and are removable like a denture, needing to cleaned and cared for by the patient.

The major function of an obturator is to block or close the opening into the nasal cavity.
It:
- stops food and drink from entering the nose space through the hole, which can be uncomfortable and embarrassing.
- helps the patient to speak normally, as they otherwise sound nasal and find difficulty in pronunciation of words.

It also:

- provides protection for healing tissues during the early stages of treatment, enabling eating and drinking normally through the mouth.
- provides support and structure for the healing tissues following surgery.
- replaces any bony structure that may have to be removed during surgery, restoring the oral cavity to its natural shape.
- provides support to the facial tissues (lips and cheeks) to give the face a natural look.
- provides teeth, if required to help:
  chewing food – mastication.
  having better speech – pronunciation.
  looking natural, improving aesthetics.
  providing confidence to carry on a normal life.

When the process of designing and manufacturing the obturator begins, we always hope to achieve the above goals. Each patient is different with unique and associated problems, and this is not always possible.

The benefit of using an obturator for the surgeon is that the surgical site can be accessed freely, and observed during healing and subsequent remodelling. It also has the advantage of making it easier to detect and react to any changes, infections or even recurrences of the tumour should this happen. Some people will go on to have the hole surgically closed, but some will have to wear an obturator for the rest of their life. Radiotherapy can play a big role in this decision, because the long-lasting effects can make reconstruction very difficult.

At first, it can seem quite daunting for patients when they find out that they have to wear one of these prostheses, but after a small amount of time, they adapt very well to their new obturator. Some patients even decide to continue wearing them as a preference to surgery, because they have learned to cope and have adapted the wearing of them into their daily lives.

We have all seen the humble denture portrayed in caricature drawings, as the joke item sitting in a glass of water by the bed of two aged citizens. We think it's funny when they pop out of people's mouths unexpectedly, following laughter or exuberant exercise. But when you understand what this small prosthesis can achieve and how much people's lives are affected by it, you begin to respect it for what it is. Thankfully, for the majority of patients, you would never be able to tell that they are even wearing an obturator.

Chapter 5

CAROL & ANN'S MEDICAL AND COMPLEMENTARY SUPPORT

This chapter is devoted to Carol and Ann's therapists. They are listed as both medical and also complementary therapists, supportive in giving help and advice.

To be able to consult the Macmillan Specialist Nurse service is a major step forward for patients. This service didn't exist in 1998.

There is an article on a GP's perspective and advice from a dentist and also a dental hygienist. Advice on swallowing and eating the right foods plays a major part in nutrition and the dietician's advice is vital. Speech therapy can be of great assistance and there are informative articles on Reiki, Hypnotherapy and Reflexology, including many other therapy treatments.

For contact details of the following therapists, please refer to *Chapter 9 Contacts and Referrals.*

MACMILLAN HEAD & NECK CLINICAL NURSE SPECIALIST

Pauline Gibbings

A Head and Neck Clinical Nurse Specialist (CNS) is one of the core members of the multidisciplinary team. At Northampton General Hospital (NGH), Macmillan adopted the role over seven years ago, giving the specialist nurse the availability of using their training and study days. Being under the umbrella of Macmillan allows the clinical nurse specialist the security and knowledge of usage of the charity's information on cancer treatments, social, financial and survivorship support.

The Macmillan Head and Neck CNS is a KEY worker for patients and carers being diagnosed and/or treated at NGH, utilising a holistic assessment showing the support and information the patient requires, as well as discussion on different treatment options. These may include: surgery, chemotherapy and radiotherapy. There is support for patients after their completed treatment with short and long-term side effects, as many patients are now surviving head and neck cancer.

As a KEY worker for patients, the Macmillan Head and Neck CNS liaises with all members of the multidisciplinary team in your care, including the consultants, maxilla facial CNS, dieticians, speech and language therapists, and many others not mentioned. The other important members are the community health professionals, including the general practitioner, district nurse and community palliative care team if required.

GENERAL PRACTITIONER

Helen Coghill
Denton Village Surgery, Northamptonshire

As a GP, I am always on the lookout for cancer. The cough could be a viral "cold", pneumonia or the first signs of a tumour; the abdominal pain may be a tummy bug or something more serious. We see thirty or more patients a day and most have minor illnesses or chronic diseases such as diabetes or heart disease which require monitoring. With ten to fifteen minutes for each consultation, there is always pressure on time.

Cancer of the oral cavity is thankfully very rare and in my career, I have seen only four in a practice of 6,000 patients. According to statistics, you are fifty times more likely to develop cancers of other areas of the body. However, there has recently been an increase in tumours associated with the Human Papillomavirus – as you may know, teenagers are now being immunised against this virus, which also causes cervical cancer, and we hope to reduce it or eventually eradicate it from the population.

Early detection of any cancer is essential, whether it is a breast lump or a suspicious mole, and I will refer anything I think is potentially a tumour to a specialist. Mouth cancer, of the type which Carol and Ann have had treated, can present to a GP as an ulcer which does not heal, an odd mark on the tongue, inner cheek or gum (dark or pale), or sometimes as a lump. Two of the cases I have seen looked like a large tonsil, but only on one side of the throat. Another presentation is simply a lump in the neck which does not go away. There can also be symptoms of tiredness or weight loss.

Dentists are very good at spotting signs of disease in the mouth – after all, they look into mouths all day! They also tend to err on the side of caution and refer anything abnormal-looking to a hospital specialist.

After treatment, there is often a long period of recovery and we are involved along with our district nursing team and sometimes Macmillan nurses. We help people recover at home with support and advice. Major surgery is often a big hurdle and the emotional wellbeing of our patients is a priority.

As Ann and Carol have proved, despite the nature of the

surgery involved, these areas of the body heal well and patients often get back to a completely normal life. I think they both show a wonderful example of how being positive aids recovery and this, of course, is true for any medical condition.

DENTAL PRACTITIONER

Dr Joanna Stock
East Park Dental Practice, Northampton

So, what are the effects of cancer treatment on the teeth and gums, and what can be done to help?

Your dentist's role may begin before the diagnosis of cancer, as a check of the soft tissues (i.e. tongue, cheeks and palate) at a routine check-up appointment. It may be the first time changes in the mouth have been noticed. Early diagnosis is important to increase the chance of success of any treatment for cancer, so if you have any concerns always see your dentist as soon as possible.

Cancer treatments including surgery or radiotherapy can have effects that potentially weaken the teeth in the long term, so it is important to take steps to keep your teeth strong. Simple steps can even be taken before the cancer treatment begins such as using a high fluoride toothpaste such as Duraphat 5000 – which is available on prescription from your dentist. Using a toothpaste that has a significantly higher fluoride content to shop-bought products, increases the benefit that fluoride offers in protecting and strengthening our teeth, which can help to reduce the risk of decay.

Initially following surgery or radiotherapy, the mouth may be very sore and swollen. Difficulties with eating could lead to a desire for simple foods that are high in sugar. As we know from being told as children, a high sugar diet increases the chance of tooth decay! When you have a sore mouth, it is very easy not to brush like you normally would. Using Chlorhexidine mouthwash such as Corsodyl or a high fluoride mouthwash like Duraphat can help to protect the teeth and gums during this time. Super soft toothbrushes are also available, such as the Tepe special care toothbrush.

Once the initial discomfort has settled following treatment, it is important to get back into good habits to care for the teeth. At this point in time, we appreciate you probably would like to avoid dental treatment where possible, but it is an ideal time for a visit to the dentist or hygienist for help and advice on a good home care routine and ways to keep the teeth and gums healthy.

After cancer treatment, some patients may encounter some new difficulties with dental treatments. One common issue is the decrease in the amount you will be able to open your jaw. This can make it more difficult for the dentist to get to the back teeth to carry out the required treatments and the muscles may become achy from holding the mouth open for a while. This may mean treatment takes a little longer than it used to. It might be worth checking when booking an appointment with the dentist that extra time has been allowed for.

For those who have undergone radiotherapy, there is a high risk of reduction in saliva production leading to a dry mouth (xerostomia). Our saliva is our natural defence against decay, so those who have a dry mouth have a greater risk of decay. Therefore, avoiding sugar and using high fluoride products is even more important.

Radiotherapy also affects your body's natural ability to heal, due to reduced blood flow in the area that was exposed to the radiation. Having a longer healing time increases your chance of infection, so we avoid tooth extractions wherever possible. If you do require an extraction, then this would usually be carried out in the maxillofacial department. Your dentist will be able to advise you what is best for you.

If you have had extensive cancer surgery, there could be an effect on the swallowing reflex. As dental procedures will generally require some form of water spray, this can add an additional complexity to treatment. However, do not worry, as with time and understanding from your dentist, most difficulties can be overcome.

Patients who have undergone cancer treatment sometimes feel, with all the other trips to the doctors and specialists, that a visit to the dentist is a low priority. However, it is more important to visit your dentist regularly to ensure a good preventative regime and catch any small problems to avoid larger prolonged treatments.

DENTAL HYGIENIST

Sharon Wright
Maxillofacial Unit, Northampton General Hospital

Sharon is a dental hygienist with many years of experience. Sharon qualified from the University of Bristol Dental Hospital in 2000, after working for several years as a qualified dental nurse in Northamptonshire. Sharon works at a number of private and NHS dental practices in the county and also works at the Maxillofacial unit as a specialist hygienist working with Oncology referrals in the field of Oral Cancer.

The dental hygienist plays an important role in meeting the unique and often challenging oral healthcare needs of patients who are impacted by cancer. Skills that hygienists already possess and new ones they can easily acquire can make the difference in the lives of these patients before, during and after cancer treatment.[1]

The initial appointment before any surgery or radiotherapy/

chemotherapy can identify any potential problems and establish the importance of good oral hygiene. This will help to minimise any potential side effects.

It is important to maintain good oral hygiene at the highest possible level during the treatment, as this can be overlooked by both the patient and other healthcare professionals whilst they are dealing with the complexity of the cancer treatment.

The hygienist will recognise each patient as an individual and adapt techniques and their treatment plan accordingly.

There are a number of common side effects of chemotherapy and radiotherapy that the patient may experience. However, I have identified the most common conditions that I observe below, with a brief description of treatment or mitigation measures.

Condition: Mucositis (ulceration and sloughing of the tissues in the mouth).
Treatment: As a result of this condition, tooth brushing may be neglected because of the sensitivity of the tissues and flavoured toothpastes sometimes cannot be tolerated. Therefore toothbrushes with a small soft textured head or single tufted toothbrushes can be recommended and unflavoured toothpastes may be beneficial.

Condition: Dry mouth (xerostomia) – a reduced quantity of saliva or changes in the saliva may be noticed. The saliva may be thickened and sticky, making swallowing difficult. These changes may make the mouth more prone to cracks and bleeding. This can make it more difficult in speaking and swallowing.
Treatment: The treatment for dry mouth would focus around effective plaque removal, application of fluorides, advice for the patient to avoid tobacco and alcohol, diet advice and to recommend

saliva substitutes. A saliva substitute is a preparation with physical and chemical properties similar to those of real saliva.

Condition: Radiation caries (dental decay) and changes in the quantity of saliva flow. In addition, dietary changes can increase the risk of caries. Teeth with exposed root surfaces of the teeth are especially susceptible.
Treatment: Good oral hygiene, fluoride toothpastes, mouthwashes and dietary factors are recommended for dental caries prevention.

Condition: Trismus (loss of elasticity of the muscles around the jaw). This limits the opening of the mouth.
Treatment: Exercises and stretching devices can be shown and used to help the patient.

In conclusion, the role of the hygienist in the treatment of oral cancer should not be underestimated. The benefits of regular appointments will ensure that the patient realises all possible benefits of dental hygiene practice, including:

- Ensuring that the patient has the maximum amount of comfort possible.
- Assisting in recovered speech.
- Assisting in the ability to eat.
- Minimising the risk of infection.

As stated, attention to detail in respect of patient oral hygiene is a key part of the treatment of oral cancer and should not be ignored, The dental hygienist can assist in the mitigation of side effects and developing a holistic care plan to support the patient through treatment and into remission and beyond.

SPEECH AND LANGUAGE THERAPY

Elaine Coker and Kelly Jackson-Waite
Northampton General Hospital

The speech and language therapists work as part of the Head and Neck multi-disciplinary team, because surgery and/or chemotherapy to the head and neck can cause changes to speech and swallowing. You may not need our services, but you will be assessed during your treatment and, if appropriate, be offered an individual therapy programme tailored to your particular needs. This may include oral swallowing exercises, dietary recommendations, and information and support for you and your family. We will work closely with the rest of the team to ensure there is an integrated approach to your treatment.

Many people ask "When will I talk properly again?" or "When will I be able to eat normal food?" Unfortunately, there is no definitive answer. So many factors play an important part in the recovery process: the extent of your particular surgery, the amount of radiotherapy you have, your healing rate, even your motivation and perseverance.

If you are having surgery, we will usually visit you on the ward after your operation to assess your speech and swallowing and offer therapy if needed. If you are having chemo-radiotherapy, we aim to meet you before the treatment to discuss the possible side effects and how these may affect your swallowing. We then see you weekly throughout the chemo-radiotherapy and for follow-up after it has finished.

If for any reason you are not seen by one of us and need advice regarding your speech or swallowing, please contact your local Adult Speech and Language Therapy Department for help.

NUTRITION

Kay Owen & Cristina Bellini,
Dieticians, Northampton General Hospital

There is a general consensus that a dietician's job is to hand out milkshakes and diet sheets. However, there is much more to dieticians than you think!

Nutrition plays a vital role in aiding recovery from surgery, chemotherapy and radiotherapy for patients with head and neck cancer. Many people feel pleased to have lost a bit of weight, but this is not the time to do it. The effects of poor nutrition are extensive, influencing speed of recovery, response to treatment, wound healing, the ability of the body to fight infection and mood.

Nutritional input varies for each person, but may include advice on nutritious high calorie and protein foods, obtaining an adequate intake when eating soft or liquidised meals, tube feeds (in hospital and home) and more specific problems such as dealing with a poor appetite, a sore mouth or taste changes. Often this involves a move away from the healthy eating principles we normally advise, to trying snacks between meals, choosing full fat and sugar versions of food and having nutritious drinks. Advice is tailored to the individual, and ongoing support for people with cancer and their families and carers is essential.

With the growth of alternative therapies over recent years, complementary and alternative therapy diets are becoming something many cancer sufferers are investigating. Some of these are safe and work well alongside standard treatments. For example, having foods containing ginger to help control nausea.

However, many alternative diets lack scientific evidence to support their claims and can be expensive to follow. They may not be safe and may possibly be harmful as they are often low in calories and protein. This may therefore exacerbate weight loss in people who are already struggling.

If you are thinking of following any alternative diets or taking any nutritional supplements, please discuss them with your doctor or dietician first.

HYPNOTHERAPY

Christine Gould MA, C.Hyp, DABCH, MABCH, MCAHyp. Registered with the Complementary and Natural Healthcare Council & Principal of The Atkinson-Ball College of Hypnotherapy and HypnoHealing

Hypnotherapy is one of the oldest and most respected medical practices known to humanity and is in essence self-hypnosis. Despite the popular misconception, subjects actually remain in control of what takes place during the session. Success is achieved when the client co-operates with an ethical hypnotherapist, who acts as a catalyst for transformational change. The skilled practitioner merely facilitates the experience in accordance with the subject's expressed outcome.

Hypnosis has been practised for thousands of years and its therapeutic use dates back to primitive times. As long ago as 350BC, Hippocrates, who was also known as 'the father of medicine', acknowledged that the source of physical disease was linked to what took place in the mind. Plato stated that, "the cure of the part should not be attempted without the treatment of the whole and therefore, if the head and body are to be well, you must begin by curing the mind".

The general consensus is that hypnosis is an altered state of consciousness and not unconsciousness. It is a natural, safe and familiar process we all experience during our lifetime and one that we pass through when drifting off to sleep and waking up. Most of us don't even realise how much time we spend, drifting in and out of hypnosis daily.

The word 'hypnosis' is derived from the Greek word 'hypnos', meaning 'sleep', which implies that in hypnosis you are asleep when in actual fact you are not. Entering hypnosis, your state of consciousness changes to feeling relaxed and drowsy, and awareness is enhanced, whilst still awake and in control of one's thoughts and actions.

Most people are familiar with 'daydreaming' and the associated feelings experienced when passing between the phase of full consciousness and semi-consciousness. Natural hypnosis is when our thoughts drift from the present reality and operate on 'autopilot'. How many times have you travelled from one place to another and can't recall part of the journey, or time has 'flown past' whilst undertaking a routine activity like washing the dishes, knitting or ironing? We still remain alert, engaged, focused and fully aware of what is going on and in an emergency can respond immediately and effectively.

A common myth about hypnosis is that it involves surrendering control and being made to do something against your will, when in fact the opposite is true. Hypnosis offers you the opportunity to tap into latent powers and exercise the ultimate in self-control.

Another myth worth dispelling is how hypnosis is depicted in movies and its association with pocket watches, trances and speaking in monotones. Contrary to this perception, in hypnosis you would never say or do anything against your personal beliefs or will.

It is also important to understand that everyone who participates in a live entertainment show is a volunteer. They have willingly elected to co-operate with the stage hypnotist and have every intention of following their suggestions. Without exception, all the volunteers are awake, aware of everything and in full control of their faculties. Should an emergency occur, they would still be responsive, alert and most probably the first people to vacate the premises if necessary.

Hypnotherapy empowers people to take responsibility for their own health and wellbeing by harnessing the power of their subconscious mind to resolve inner conflict and change existing or negative behaviour patterns.

An experienced hypnotherapist will skilfully guide the client into hypnosis by facilitating access to their subconscious mind, which is the seat of all emotional and behavioural problems. Working co-operatively, changes can be made in accordance with the client's desired outcomes. In effect, making the changes is similar to updating the programmes on a computer or reorganising your filing system.

This dynamic therapy can be considered a type of preventative medicine, recognised for its value in the treatment of many conditions. Acknowledging that the mind and body are closely related, the medical professions are increasingly recommending hypnotherapy and self-hypnosis to address a variety of behavioural, emotional and health problems.

Hypnotherapy is regularly used to manage acute and chronic pain, for burns, asthma, migraine, hay fever, irritable bowel syndrome and with cancer patients to relieve the side effects of chemotherapy or radiotherapy. It can also help in the relief of many psychosomatic disorders, as well as maximising potential in artistic, creative and sporting fields.

HypnoHealing is a specialised method that addresses health and physical problems. It works on the basis that the mind heals the body. Positive changes lead to favourable outcomes and when the mind believes, the body responds accordingly. Only graduates of the world-renowned Atkinson-Ball College are trained in this technique.

Hypnotherapy is not just about problems. It is about achieving effortless change and getting in touch with why you are the way you are and becoming the person you really want to be.

People who become conversant with techniques for self-hypnosis and take time to incorporate it into their daily lives, find the benefits tremendous. By actively taking personal responsibility for your own wellbeing, deep states of relaxation can be achieved. This leads to enhanced personal awareness, boosts vitality, promotes self-healing, focuses attention, and harnesses inner resources for accelerated potential in every area of life. Like any skill, it requires practice and when you have mastered it, you have a resource that is yours forever.

Answers to some frequently asked questions

What is hypnosis?
A state of relaxation in which the client is very aware of what is going on and is in complete control at all times. While in hypnosis, you would never say or do anything that you wouldn't normally do, whereas people who participate in live shows have volunteered to behave in an uninhibited manner.

Can anyone be hypnotised?
Yes, if they want to be.

Will I be asleep?
No. You will be aware of what is going on all the time and just feel relaxed.

Can I be forced to do anything against my will?
Emphatically – NO! The client is always in total control.

Are there any harmful side effects?
Definitely not, because hypnosis is a natural phenomenon we all experience every day.

How does hypnotherapy differ from other therapies?
Many therapies are conducted on a conscious level, whereas in hypnosis you bypass the conscious mind. This allows direct contact with your subconscious mind, where existing or negative behaviour patterns can be changed and inner conflict resolved.

How many visits will I need?
Three to four sessions are generally sufficient and for more deep-rooted problems, possibly five or six.

Christine Gould runs a thriving private practice in the heart of England and has worked within the National Health Service for over twenty years. Originally, she formed part of a multidisciplinary team at the Pain Relief Clinic. However, in recent years, she spends most of her time helping oncology patients and young people attending the Children's Outpatients Department.

REIKI

Christine Gould
International Reiki Master Teacher

The power of loving touch is a meaningful source of comfort and connection with our loved ones. When we reach out and touch another with our Reiki-empowered hands, they become a potent resource for stimulating the body's infinite healing capacity.

Dr Mikao Usui rediscovered this ancient tradition of energy transmission through the hands over a century ago. He was a distinguished Japanese scholar of comparative religions, searching to find out how the ancients healed. After many years, he came across a formula in Sanskrit texts and, to explore its potential, decided to climb Mount Kurama and spend three weeks in quiet contemplation and meditation. On his return journey back to Kyoto, circumstances led Dr Usui to apply the techniques he had intuitively perceived. From firsthand personal experience, he gained confirmation of its validity and named the system Reiki.

Even though Reiki, pronounced 'ray-key', is a Japanese word, it is believed this modality originated in Tibet. The syllables each have a definition; 'rei' means 'universal' and 'ki' denotes 'life energy'.

Eastern philosophies have a broad vocabulary for discussing the vital life forces that permeate and nourish all living forms. Ancient Chinese use the concept of Chi or Qi, whereas prana is used by the Hindus, pneuma by the Greeks and ka by the Egyptians.

Reiki is independent of all conventional religions, making it compatible with people's beliefs regardless of age, culture, doctrine or status. Hence, it is available to everyone. There are no prerequisites or academic qualifications necessary to train as a Reiki channel. Its simplicity and accessibility is demonstrated by the fact that children as young as seven years of age may attend the class, at the discretion of the Reiki Master Teacher.

Undertaking Reiki training is the easiest way of harnessing the universal life force energy, which, in essence, is purely and simply unconditional love. Students are required to have four 'energy transfers' or 'attunements' in order to channel the external and additional flow of energy. These sacred processes make this modality unique and are the hallmark of Reiki. They are similar to retuning a television from analogue to digital frequencies for clearer, stronger signals.

Reiki is instantly accessible and activated by engaging one or both hands on anything living, whether yourself, others, animals or plants. It does not require any regular exercise routines, postures, specific breathing patterns or mantras that tai chi, qui gong and yoga do. As Reiki flows through a practitioner, the brain wave patterns change from beta to alpha cycles, which is the natural rhythm of the universe and similar to a meditative or hypnotic state. All bodily functions slow down, including the ageing process, whereas the biological intelligence that promotes the body's resources to heal is amplified.

When practising Reiki, it has been scientifically demonstrated on monitoring equipment that oxygen in the haemoglobin increases by up to thirty per cent. Elevated levels of oxygen in the blood, tissues and cells improve the regenerative processes, accelerate healing, relieve pain and alleviate stress. This makes Reiki beneficial for anyone experiencing health issues.

Reiki is regularly used as a complement to traditional medicine and natural therapies. Regardless of whether you are fit and well, have a health issue or challenge in your life, Reiki provides a complete system of self-healing that can be readily implemented at any time. It is far more than a physical healing modality, because it brings into balance all four aspects of self; the mental, spiritual, emotional and physical. With the appropriate resources, the body is capable of being restored to its original healthy blueprint.

Many people report feeling a deep sense of relaxation, warmth, tingling or chill during a Reiki treatment, whereas others experience subtle sensations or maybe nothing at all. The effects may be felt physically or they may bring about a change of attitude, inspirational thought, creative insight, or solutions to challenging situations. It reduces tension and discomfort, whilst inducing inner calm and renewed enthusiasm for life.

It is a valuable first-aid tool which can be used at any time, whether at home, work or leisure. In an emergency, there is evidence of rapid physical healing – manifested by burns that do not blister – pain relief, a reduction of swelling, the cessation of bleeding and bruises that tend to fade overnight. An additional bonus is the ability to maintain a sense of calm and emotional stability.

In accordance with Dr Usui's teachings, there are only two levels of Reiki at practitioner level. In both cases, direct hand to body contact is made, making this literally a hands-on-healing modality. Using the advanced procedures, the physical body is often substituted by what is called a proxy. Reiki is the only system of self-healing that does not require a practitioner. Graduates can treat themselves effectively, just as if another practitioner was treating them.

Reiki Level I – Basic Training Course

This seminar usually takes place on Friday evening, Saturday and Sunday. Each student receives four energy procedures or 'attunements', they learn the twelve basic hand positions; how to conduct a self-treatment; how to work on another person, in a group situation, with animals, plants and in an emergency.

Included in the curriculum are powerful metaphysical insights about the cause and effect of illness and personal circumstances. These illustrate how the body is a metaphor for the psyche, and how every condition and situation has a deep and significant meaning.

This personally empowering seminar also includes the history, philosophy and principles of Reiki, leading to:

- Improved Communication
- Heightened Self-Awareness
- Enhanced Relationships
- Increased Self-Confidence
- Personal Growth
- Metaphysical Understanding
- Stress Reduction
- Certification
- Course Manual
- Postgraduate Support

There is no need to attend regular classes, have any top-ups or to make further financial investments. Graduates have the privilege to review other Reiki I seminars at no additional cost.

Reiki Level II – Advanced Training Course

This is an optional three-day seminar when students learn three symbols to project the energy over distance for absent healing, or work directly on themselves and others. There are two further attunements, which promote an increased flow and potency of energy. An additional bonus is the enhancement of intuitive and telepathic abilities.

Christine Gould undertook a five-year apprenticeship, which entailed travelling and teaching globally, to become the second Reiki Master Teacher initiated by Barbara McGregor (Aus). Years later, she studied with John Harvey Gray (USA) to qualify as a Reiki Master Teacher. This makes her fifth in line to Dr Usui, with possibly the clearest lineage in the UK.

SPIRITUAL HEALING

Christine Gould

Spiritual Healing is an ancient therapy that has been practised throughout history. Natural or Hands-on Healing, together with available herbs, is all that our ancient civilisations could use to calm fevers and ailments.

Many people confuse Spiritual Healing and Spiritualism, when in fact they are not the same. Spiritual Healing is not connected to any specific religion and is compatible with all beliefs. The word 'spiritual' refers to the quality of spirituality (or self) implicit in the healing process.

Spirit is within people and animals, too. It is part of us that makes us unique – the inner self, which reflects our vitality and state of mental, emotional and physical wellbeing. When reference is made to someone or an animal being 'high spirited', this suggests they are in a state of high vitality whereas the opposite, 'low spirited', indicates lack of vitality.

The essence of Spiritual Healing is that practitioners tap into the universal life force or divine spiritual energy and act as a channel for the flow of healing energy to the recipient. The aim is to enhance balance, thereby encouraging the body to self-heal, utilising its own natural resources, and become whole and well. Healing works on every aspect of the person to promote harmony of mind, body and spirit.

Practitioners channel universal life force energy through the hands to those in need and elect to receive Spiritual Healing. The healer will either make direct contact with the person or place their hands close to, but not touching, the physical body. Energy may be channelled to a specific area or towards the whole body. It may be experienced in various ways such as heat, coolness, warmth, tingling, or a relaxed and comfortable feeling. Each person is unique and the sensations can vary for each treatment.

Several forms of healing are available under the auspices of the National Health Service in many hospitals, GP's surgeries and clinics. It is considered a safe and beneficial form of therapy, irrespective of the medical diagnosis.

Spiritual Healing is completely natural and has no side effects. It may be given for any illness, psychological, emotional or physical condition, and is regularly used alongside conventional medicine. As well as its value in relieving pain and restoring the body to its natural balanced state, people have reported improved attitudes, clarity of thought and a better quality of daily life.

All types of healing are beneficial and usually the process is progressive. Several treatments may be necessary before a change becomes obvious. Although many spontaneous recoveries are made, the benefits can sometimes be subtle and not in the way expected. Some may develop a different outlook on life, regardless of their mental or physical condition, and start to appreciate what they can do rather than what they can't. If someone is empowered to cope with their circumstances, their quality of life is enhanced.

Healing is helpful before and after major surgery, serious injury, trauma or with the after effects of chemotherapy and radiotherapy. It also boosts the immune system, thus promoting feelings of improved wellbeing. When working with the terminally ill, healing helps induce a sense of peace to them and their loved ones.

Distant and absent healing is also reported to be very effective. Dedicated practitioners will regularly spend time channelling healing energy by use of meditation techniques to those in need, regardless of whether the person is in the same room or miles away, with similar positive responses.

The beneficial effects of Spiritual Healing for animals are well documented; however, none of the techniques should be applied without obtaining the permission of a vet.

CYMATHERAPY

Christine Gould

Cymatherapy is a combination of sound healing and magnetic therapy dedicated to restoring optimal good health and wellbeing. These combined cutting-edge techniques are produced by the Cyma 1000. This state-of-the-art, acoustic instrument emits sounds, programmed with biological messages that the body assimilates, to support its innate healing ability.

The power of sound has been an integral part of ancient cultures through religion, magic or healing since time began. It was fundamental to all primitive societies, either as chanting, drumming, toning, harmonic and choral singing, as lullabies working songs, or to serenade a loved one.

In society today, sound represents different things to each of us and for many people it is a natural accompaniment to daily life. It is used to please and entertain, modify moods and control feelings, advance spiritual development and enhance awareness. There are many advantages when it is used with wisdom, knowledge and understanding. It can create a sense of balance and harmony, calm us, accelerate our energies or assist meditation.

Scientists recognise that the human body is a highly structured complex of rhythms and cyclic vibrations. When all aspects are collaboratively operating in harmony – including heartbeat, respiratory rhythms, blood pressure, pulse rate, hormonal levels, tissues and cells – then good health abounds. Similar to an orchestra; when all musicians play in harmony, the result is pleasing. Conversely, the effect of dissonant sounds is unfavourable to the ear.

During the past few years, the power of sound, as a therapeutic modality, has increased especially in the field of medicine. Music therapy is regularly used to reduce stress, for pain management, in dentistry, delivery rooms and operating theatres, when dealing with the elderly and with those experiencing special needs and emotional issues. Ultrasound is another example. Healthcare practitioners regularly prescribe ultrasound to diagnose tumours, clean wounds, pulverise kidney stones and alleviate pain in sore muscles and backs.

All sounds have the ability to transmit energy through a process known as 'resonance'. Every part of the anatomy, the cells, organs and tissues have their own natural resonance or frequency. Each responds positively to sounds that vibrate in harmony with them. The opposite occurs when discordant sounds are perceived, which can lead to harmful results.

Building on the science of Cymatics, forty years of cutting-edge research has culminated with technology taking energetic sound healing to a new level. Cymatics is the study of wave phenomena pioneered by the Swiss medical doctor and natural scientist, Hans Jenny. He spent fourteen years conducting experiments about how sound manifests into form. The shapes and patterns that emerged using sand, powders, mercury, etc. from the effects of tones, music and vocal sound were filmed and recorded.

The implications of Dr. Jenny's work for healing and vibrational medicine were vast. If sounds could change substances, what effect would they have on our cellular structure? This inspired others, including English osteopath Peter Guy Manners, to explore how cells in an unhealthy body differ from the cells in a vibrant healthy one. It was from this research that Cymatherapy has evolved.

Cymatherapy delivers natural sound frequencies that restore unhealthy cells to their original healthy resonance. This vibrational technique aims to transform disturbed inner rhythms using sound pulsations transmitted by a hand-held machine. It is placed over the area of the body to be treated and frequencies matching the cells in a healthy body are emitted.

The Cyma 1000 instrument offers a wide range of harmonious codes that produce precise combinations of frequencies and audible sound waves, along with magnetic therapy, to synchronise the cells back to a natural healthy state of vibrational resonance.

The audible harmonious frequencies are combined with the Chinese Five-Element theory, the Meridian system, Chakras, energetic stem cells and hormones. Together, they create an integrated mapping system of energetic healing for the sound pathways in the body.

This unique and revolutionary system works effectively on both animals and people. In America, it is regularly used with horses and household pets.

Cymatherapy may be supportive in rebalancing the dissonant energies related to: addictions, anger, arthritis, irritable bowel syndrome, depression, digestive problems, dystonia, phobias, physical injuries, aches and pains and much more.

The Cymatherapy vibrational techniques have been reported to be effective for facial rejuvenation, which is similar to non-surgical face-lifts. Many practitioners in America specialise in this procedure.

Case Studies

Cricket Phobia: Budding cricketer George, aged fourteen, flinched every time the ball was bowled towards him. This was becoming an increasing concern for the county coach and his father. George was also struggling academically and so during the first session of Cymatherapy, a variety of codes were used to address these issues. Upon his return three weeks later, George reported that all his anxieties had subsided and he could confidently address the ball. His father declared how his school performance had improved and that George had come third out of his year group of 150 students in the cross-country sports event. Somewhat perplexed by these improvements, his father is delighted that George's potential has increased.

Back Problem: Orthopaedic Surgeon Natasha, in her mid-thirties, had suffered with low back pain since the birth of her youngest child four years earlier. During her lunch hour, she came across a demonstration of the Cyma 1000 taking place in the local hospital. Curious to experience this new technology, she asked for a demonstration. After ten minutes, her bleep sounded and Natasha said she had to leave. Standing up, her keys fell to the floor and automatically she reached down to retrieve them. Natasha was shocked, yet astonished that she achieved this with such ease and wondered how the pain had totally vanished.

Bursitis: Kellie had a limited range of movement in her left arm and experienced pain when lying in bed. Applying the applicator over the site for fifteen minutes relieved the discomfort, and Kellie was able to raise her arm above her head for the first time in four months. A second session resulted in complete restoration of movement, enabling her to resume riding her beloved horse with confidence.

HOLISTIC MASSAGE

Kay Hughes

It is said the first sense we develop when born is touch and it is the last of the senses to leave us when we die.

Massage is about touch. It is a time for the client to shut out all external distractions and focus on themselves.

Now, they are truly free! Physically listening to their own bodies. Maybe emotionally trusting the process of the massage and the support of the therapist to let go of their emotions safely. Mentally, it creates space to clear the mind and feel more energised, refreshed and recharged. This holistic approach of balancing mind, body and emotional states is very powerful on the journey of living and self-healing.

Massage has many techniques and an experienced therapist will choose what is appropriate for the client after the consultation, really listening to what the client feels and wants the massage to do for them.

Massage has many benefits and is available in many forms – from gentle Swedish massage (tender loving care); deeper tissue remedial massage to ease areas of discomfort and enhance the lymphatic system to be more efficient (or, as I say, 'to clear the plumbing'); or working on the nervous system by gentle pressure along the spinal column to release the muscles and allow oxygen to go to the cells.

Massage is a truly beautiful experience. It is holistic, treating the whole person and not just the condition, and has physical well-being and physiological benefits. It is a sacred safe space built on trust between client and therapist, allowing the healing and wellbeing process to be stimulated. It is a most important time to be yourself as a human-being and not a human-doing.

REFLEXOLOGY

Joan Innes MAR BTAA Cert Ed
Moulton Therapies

Reflexology is a non-intrusive complementary therapy; a reflexologist works on hands or feet, feeling for reflexes. Some of the earliest evidence of Reflexology dates back to ancient Egypt, but the treatment we are familiar with today was bought to the UK by Doreen Bayly. An American Ear, Nose and Throat specialist, Dr. William Fitzgerald "discovered" zone therapy around 1909. He used the principle to anaesthetise his patients locally during surgery by applying pressure to fingers, mouth and toes. Developing this theory, Eunice Ingham created Reflexology – later learnt by Doreen Bayly, who bought it to the UK in the 1960s and started the first Reflexology Training School in Great Britain.

Reflexology is a sequenced application of finger and thumb pressure to the feet and hands to stimulate the natural healing processes of the body. Reflexologists believe that the points on the feet and hands relate to specific organs, functions and parts of the body.

Reflexology can be given to anyone at any age; however, there are occasionally times when it is not suitable to provide treatment.

A detailed medical history is taken upon the first visit to a reflexologist, and the feet are examined. The reflexologist works fingers and thumbs over the soles of the feet or palms of the hands, feeling for reflexes that are revealing imbalances in the body. The treatment should not be uncomfortable to even sensitive feet.

Each body reacts differently to treatment and experiences vary, but usually a sense of deep relaxation and sense of wellbeing is felt. Increased relaxation may help to allow the body to heal health conditions. Complementary therapies can fit into all lifestyles and can be part of an individual's coping strategy. Professional reflexologists demonstrate they have met the strictest standards of Reflexology practice and are committed to continually develop their skills.

AROMATHERAPIST AND REFLEXOLOGIST

Jo Wiles

Reflexology is a complementary therapy, which uses reflex points on the feet – the body being mapped out on the feet – to assist the rebalancing of the body. It is an ancient therapy which is still in demand now and very many people feel great benefits from the therapy.

In the context of working with people on their cancer journey and also those who are caring for people on this journey, Reflexology has a great deal to offer as a therapy. It helps to re-balance the energies needed for the body to heal itself, but it also relaxes and de-stresses the person receiving the reflexology. This can, in turn, help give the person a moment of relief and escape from the mental exhaustion of the situation they find themselves in. It can have a positive effect on their sleep as well, giving them a little more energy to cope with the symptoms of treatment.

Reflexology is usually carried out on the feet and certain reflexes may be sensitive when they are worked – however, people do still find it relaxing. Very occasionally, the therapy is not suitable for a particular person. The pressure that the therapist uses when they work on the person's reflexes is firm and therefore very rarely is ticklish feet an issue. The hands can be worked on if the feet are not able to be treated.

I am a full-time therapist based in Studio 53 in Duston, Northampton and I have also worked, on a voluntary basis, with people on their cancer journey through the Dunstone Bennett Suite, since its inception. I hope it will carry on being well used in the future by all those who wish to use it.

TRANSFERENCE HEALING

Sandy Reygan
Where does it all come from? Alexis Cartwright who lives in Sydney, Australia is the channel and founder of Transference healing® who holds the technology of this modality.

It will activate and template a unique healing process. Transference Healing® is a seventh dimensional frequency healing and ascension process. It works with the light-body and creates alchemy. We are currently evolving along with the planet and, in turn, viruses, illness and symptoms are changing. Therefore, our methods of healing need to change in order to remain effective, and to be able to maintain wellness at this time in our evolution.

We need to regularly clean, realign and balance all of our energy bodies. Transference Healing® works on all levels – physical, mental, emotional and spiritual – to allow you to achieve alignment, balance and wellness, at the same time as accelerating your spiritual growth.

It is suitable for all ages, conditions and illnesses. It is very effective and is easily incorporated into your life. Experiencing a one-to-one Transference Healing® can be a profound and enlightening experience. We begin with a brief discussion and highlight any intentions for the healing. We then allow the heart to be receptive to healing and light, gently shifting into a fifth dimensional space, channeling both alchemical and light-body procedures. To complete the session, an intuitive reading and light-body essence help you hold and integrate the frequency.

If you feel drawn to receive Transference Healing® but not in person, I can offer absentee sessions which are extremely powerful. I connect to your energy and call you into my healing space and work as if you were present in the room. You will then receive a recorded personal reading emailed as an mp3 or posted CD recording, a posted light-body essence and an option to speak with me by Skype or telephone after your healing.

You will find a Transference Healing® session to be very relaxing, heartfelt and a genuinely healing experience.

HEALTH AND BEAUTY

Michele Dupuy-Sherratt

I am Michele Dupuy-Sherratt, a fully qualified therapist running my own business, and met Ann Bennett seven years prior to the beginnings of the Dunstone Bennett Complementary Centre. We first met when Ann became a client and during preceding years, we have become close friends. I had no hesitation in offering my therapy services voluntarily at the Dunstone Bennett Centre (DB) when it opened at the Cripps in October 2009.

I have been actively involved at the centre ever since, offering the centre's clients a range of therapies including body massage and Indian head massage, together with a range of beauty treatments. I am able to offer advice and treatments to men and women of all ages via the centre now located on Billing Road.

A focus of my treatments is to offer practical solutions to skin issues. Ongoing medical treatments can result in changes in the skin, skin texture and tone, as well as changes in hair texture and colour. I offer advice on skin care, offering facials, eyebrow tinting and general make-up selection and application.

Initially, clients are both nervous and apprehensive. Even though the treatments offer practical and therapeutic solutions, these go much further in restoring confidence in the client. These treatments are also available to family members and carers, all of whom need the same support and care.

HAIR AND BEAUTY

Deborah Smith
Hair and Beauty co-ordinator, Hair and Beauty Service

The Hair and Beauty Service's main aim is to support and advise men and women who are receiving cancer treatment, who as a result can/will experience hair loss.

You will be referred to the Hair and Beauty Service, by either your consultant or specialist nurse, prior to receiving chemotherapy/radiotherapy treatment and before your hair loss occurs.

You may be eligible to use the cool cap system which can significantly reduce the amount of hair loss that chemotherapy causes, but it is only available for use with certain types of chemotherapy drugs. This will be discussed with you if you are a candidate for its use.

You will be issued (free of charge if you are an NHS Patient) with a high quality modern hairpiece.

The hairpieces are available in many different colours and styles and a large selection of headwear and accessories are available for you to purchase if you require.

Make-up advice and demonstrations are also given, which can include the application of false eyelashes.

I am available for you to contact at any stage of your treatment and can offer advice on all aspects of your hair loss, hair regrowth, hair management and colouring. A wig cutting/hair cutting service is also available.

You will be seen consistently throughout your cancer treatment and you will be treated holistically with empathy and with an understanding of your situation and concerns.

The hair and beauty service is a valued service which provides help and advice throughout your cancer journey.

Quotes from patients:-

"You were wonderful on my visits. You were understanding of my feelings and emotions and treated me with great kindness and care."

"You made a difficult time so much easier."

"You provide a very caring, sensitive, professional and supportive service. It really made a difference."

Chapter 6

RECIPES FOR MOUTH CANCER PATIENTS

TIPS

Nutrition is the key to good health and vitality. To regain your full strength and optimum health, you need to eat well.

The best sources of protein are: MEAT, FISH, EGGS, CHEESE, MILK, YOGHURT and SOYA.

Bread, biscuits, rice, flour, cream, cereals, potato, nuts, chocolate, peas and lentils also contain some protein. Protein provides materials for tissue repair and growth.

The most concentrated sources of energy are fat, butter and oils. These can be used in cooking, on bread, vegetables, etc. Sugars, glucose, jam, honey and Lucozade are another valuable energy source.

An adequate intake of protein, calories and vitamin C is important. A high calorie intake is essential with a fluid diet to maintain body weight and provide energy for building new tissues.

Vitamin C is essential for healing and the health of skin and gums. Fluids rich in vitamin C are fresh, canned or frozen orange and grapefruit juice, Ribena and Rosehip Syrup. Take one glass of a vitamin C rich drink every day.

Vegetables should be part of a balanced diet. Supplementary drinks such as milk shakes, Build Up and Complan or Fortisips, which are drunk between meals, contribute substantial amounts of both protein and energy. These can also be used to replace meals when you have lost your appetite or are feeling unwell.

Try to have three good meals a day and at least one pint of milk each day. Cook food well and mash with fork or put in liquidiser with plenty of sauce or gravy to aid swallowing until chewing improves. Liquid feeds should be taken through a straw or sipped from a spoon or glass.

Take small frequent meals to ensure an adequate intake of calories and protein.

Some ideas:

- Liquidise or sieve soups – add milk or milk powder or double cream.
- Liquidise ordinary meals (meat, vegetables and potato), then mix with soup, gravy or milk until the required consistency has been obtained.
- Try baby foods.
- Oxo, Bovril and Marmite can be used as flavourings or mixed with boiled water as a drink.
- Use prepared sauce mixes and cook-in sauces.

Milk puddings and custard may be managed if diluted with milk. They may be sweetened with glucose or sugar and fortified with milk powder, Complan, Build Up, evaporated milk or double cream to provide extra protein and calories.

Yoghurts, if necessary, can be thinned down with milk and taken as a drink, flavoured with pureed fruit or seedless jam. Ice cream and jelly are another alternative.

In the early days of recovery, I found sauces invaluable and I still do. Soups are important and nutritious and organic soups are particularly good. Thin soups are perhaps easier when drunk from a mug. Pureed soups are excellent, especially if thick like a potage. It's often easier if soups have been liquidised, as there is less chance of coughing and choking.

Try and use vegetables in season e.g. broccoli, tomatoes, spinach, garlic, sweet potatoes, potatoes, beans, peas, cauliflower, red peppers, aubergines, courgettes, carrots and greens – to name but a few. They are good if steamed on top or baked in the oven. A sauce can be added to help swallowing. Eggs can be scrambled, poached or softly boiled and mashed up with a little butter, made into an omelette or eggy bread.

Recipe for eggy bread: Mix whole eggs and milk and season to taste. Whisk together with a fork. Dip slices of bread mixture and coat. Fry both sides gently in olive oil or butter until golden brown.

Eating a variety of food remains important in order to provide a balanced diet.

Other tips and suggestions:

- Lentils and pulses can be added to dishes.
- Rice may be difficult for some.
- Mashed potato can be used as a carrier with other savoury foods. This has now become a major part of my staple diet.

- Lots of sauces and gravies.
- Pineapple sucked in the mouth very gently helps to produce saliva and also fight off bad bacteria.
- Plenty of liquids like cold water and milk. I always carry a bottle of water with me, jokingly referred to as my *gin* bottle.
- Porridge or Ready Brek are excellent for breakfast.
- Mashed bananas.
- Stewed fruits, e.g. apples, pears, plums and gooseberry fool.
- Yoghurts and smoothies.

Hunger can be a challenge to overcome. Here are some suggestions to *fill the gap:*

- Porridge with active manuka honey has very good healing properties.
- Pureed dates.
- Pure chocolate melted in milk, or any type of alternative milk or water.
- Pureed fruit with ice cream, yoghurt or sorbet.
- Various fruit jellies.
- Pureed carrot.
- Salmon mashed with a sauce.
- Minced chicken, turkey or lamb.
- Pilchards and sardines.
- Mashed potato, sweet potato and avocado.
- Add eggs to dishes for extra protein.

Additional useful tips

- Use Bio Oil to help with skin scarring

- Arnica & Paracetamol for bruising and pain.
- Movicol for any tummy problems after surgery and medication which can be requested through your doctor

JUICES

(Metric measures are rounded up to match imperial measures)

The following juices contain beta-carotene, vitamins C and E, and Selenium, and can be drunk on a regular basis to provide all-round goodness – but don't forget to keep eating whole fruit and vegetables, too. You can find high quantities of beta-carotene in whole oranges and vegetables, as well as dark green leafy vegetables.

Each recipe makes approximately one 8 fluid oz (230 ml) glass of juice. Adults can drink up to three glasses daily, but do vary the juice combinations for maximum benefit. Drink diluted if you prefer. Juice each ingredient and then blend using a spoon.

1. 2 large carrots
    1 mango

2. 1 medium canteloupe melon

3. 3 large carrots
    6 large spinach leaves

4. 1 nectarine
    1 peach

5. ¼ sweet potato
    2 tomatoes
    2 large carrots

6. A handful of watercress
    2 large carrots
    ¼ red bell pepper

BERRY BOOSTER

175 g (6 oz) raspberries
175 g (6 oz) blackberries
Sparkling mineral water

Process all the fruit in the juicer. Add the mineral water to taste.

SURPRISE JUICE

6 apricots
6 lychees
2 apples

Halve the apricots and remove stones. Peel the lychees and remove stones. Cut the apples into wedges. Process all the fruit in the juicer.

WONDER JUICE

5 carrots
1 beetroot
4 watercress sprigs
1 clove garlic, peeled

Trim the carrots. Cut the beetroot into wedges. Process all the vegetables in the juicer.

CABBAGE JUICE

4 spinach leaves
4 carrots
7.5 cm (3 in) wedge of green cabbage
¼ potato scrubbed

Form the spinach leaves into balls. Trim the carrots. Process all the vegetables in the juicer.

PINEAPPLE JUICE

2 pineapple rounds – 2.5 cm (1 in) thick
2 apples
1 mango

Remove the outer skin from the pineapple and cut the flesh into strips. Cut the apples into wedges. Peel the mango and remove the stone. Process all the fruit in the juicer.

ELSA'S FRUIT SMOOTHIE

Take a selection of fresh soft fruits such as mango, banana, peach or nectarine.

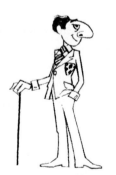

Liquidise with just enough fresh orange and apple juice to produce a thin puree.

Combine with a carton of Actimel, which sweetens and reduces acidity as well as making the drink easier to swallow.

TIP! If you can't be bothered to peel any fruit, just combine a commercial organic smoothie with Actimel for the same result.

PEGGY'S SOUPS:

CREOLE SOUP

1 large onion	50 g (1 oz) butter
1 small tin pimentos	2 tbsp plain flour
1 tin tomatoes	1 tsp tomato puree
Paprika to taste	1.2 l (2 pints) chicken stock
1 dstsp horseradish sauce	1 tbsp cream
(optional)	

Chop onion finely and fry gently in butter until soft.

Add chopped peppers and cook 1 – 2 minutes.

Stir in flour and cook 1 – 2 minutes.

Add stock, tomatoes, tomato puree and seasoning.

Bring to boil and simmer 10 – 15 minutes.

Blend and then pass through a vegetable mill.

Adjust seasoning and add horseradish if desired.

Add a tablespoon of cream.

TIP! This might be a little too spicy for some people. It is also possible to use a liquidiser to blend the above ingredients.

AVOCADO AND SPINACH SOUP

2 avocado pears	½ litre chicken stock
150 ml (¼ pint) cream or yoghurt	Juice and rind of 1 lemon
300 g (12 oz) frozen or blanched	Seasoning to taste
Spinach(well drained)	

Scoop out avocado flesh.
Place in blender with rest of ingredients.
Blend until smooth.
Chill.

TIP! To keep colour of spinach, leave in fridge to last moment and serve in cold dishes.

POTAGE BONNE FEMME

750 g (1 ½ lbs) potatoes
50 – 70 g (2 – 3 oz) butter
Seasoning to taste
3 large leeks, sliced
2 litres (3 pints) water or light chicken stock

To finish:
2 – 4 tbsp cream
Parsley or chervil(chopped) and chives
Nut of butter

Melt butter in a large pan.
Add sliced leeks and cook gently until soft and shining.
Peel and dice potatoes. Add to leeks and cook for 2 – 3 minutes.
Pour on stock, season, bring to boil and cook gently for 25 – 30 minutes.
Pass through the coarse and then fine plate of the vegetable mill. (DO NOT PUT IN LIQUIDISER.)
Reheat, adjust seasoning and add butter, herbs and cream just before serving.

POTAGE AU CELERI

2 hearts of celery
75 g (3 oz) butter
150 ml (¼ pint) single cream

2 large potatoes, thinly sliced
2 pints vegetable or light chicken
stock

Cook celery gently in 50 g (2 oz) butter for 5 minutes.

Add the potatoes, stirring occasionally, and cook for 5 minutes.

Add the stock, bring to the boil, season and simmer for 20 – 30 minutes.

Pass mixture through a vegetable mill into a clean pan.

Reheat and adjust seasoning.

Just before serving, add cream and whisk in 25g (1 oz) butter.

BUTTERNUT SQUASH AND SWEET POTATO SOUP

Donated by Joy Ball
serves 4

1 butternut squash, peeled, deseeded and diced
1 sweet potato, peeled and diced
2 carrots, trimmed, peeled and sliced
1 fennel bulb, trimmed and chopped (optional)

6 shallots, peeled and finely sliced
1 garlic clove, peeled and chopped
4 tbsp chopped fresh parsley
1 bunch radishes, trimmed
4-6 tbsp pumpkin seeds (optional)
1 wheat-free vegetable stock cube

Bring a large pan half-filled with water to the boil. Add the squash, sweet potato, carrots, fennel, shallots and stock cube. Bring to the boil, then lower the heat and simmer for 10 – 12 minutes.

Remove from the heat and add garlic.

Allow to cool, then strain the vegetables into a large bowl to keep the stock.

Add half the stock to the vegetables and blend in a food processor or with a hand-held blender to desired consistency.

Reheat the soup gently, adding more of the reserved stock if necessary.

Divide between warmed soup bowls and serve garnished with the parsley, radishes and pumpkin seeds.

VEGETABLE SOUP

Donated by Manjit Ohri

1 onion

1 carrot

Small bundle broccoli

2 tbsp red lentils

1.2 l (2 pints) boiling water

Vegetable oil for frying

1 potato

1 tsp mixed herbs

1 vegetable stock cube

Salt and pepper to taste

Chop and fry onion until brown.

Add mixed herbs, chopped vegetables and lentils.

Mix stock cube in boiling water and pour over the vegetables.

Cover and simmer until the vegetables are cooked.

Take off the heat and blend.

Season to taste.

CELERY SOUP

Donated by Frankie Button

1 tbsp olive oil	Seasoning
Half a bay leaf	1 onion finely chopped
1 litre (1 ½ pints) chicken or	1 head of celery finely chopped
Vegetable stock	Pinch of mixed herbs

Heat the oil in a large saucepan, add the onions and soften without browning. Add celery, stock, bay leaf and seasoning. Cover and simmer for about 30 minutes or until vegetables are soft. This soup may be liquidised or not, as preferred.

LENTIL SOUP

Donated by Frankie Button

1 tbsp sunflower oil	2 onions chopped
3 carrots chopped	1 tbsp tomato puree
1 litre (1 ½ pints) vegetable stock	Bouquet garni
225 grams (9 oz) red lentils	3 rashers streaky bacon chopped
2 sticks celery chopped	(omit for vegetarians)

Heat the oil in saucepan and gently sauté the bacon, celery, carrots and onions for 4-5 minutes. Add other ingredients, bring to the boil and simmer gently for 1 hour or until lentils are soft. Puree or liquidise the soup and gently reheat.

COUNTRY VEGETABLE SOUP

Donated by Erika Takacs
serves 4

500 g (1 lb) carrots
500 g (1 lb) French beans
500 g (1 lb) Kholrabi
1 lb parsnips
1 lb small onions
1 clove garlic

500 g (1 lb) potatoes (optional)
Roux sauce:
2 to 3 tbsp oil
2 tbsp plain flour (or rice flour)
1 tsp red paprika

Cut all vegetables into little cubes.

Cook all ingredients in a stockpot until tender.

Season to taste and liquidise or leave chunky.

Heat oil in pan and fry flour until golden brown.

Take off the heat and add red paprika.

Mix roux well and add to soup.

Stir well and bring to boil, adding water according to thickness required.

May be served with shell pasta or croutons.

CHICKEN AND VEGETABLE SOUP

Donated by Erika Takacs

2 nice pieces of chicken breast
500 g (1 lb) carrots, sliced into round circles
250 g (½ lb) parsnips, sliced into round circles
1 small onion (use whole)
3 bay leaves

1.8 litres (3 pints) water
A little milk
A good handful of fresh parsley or
1 tbsp dry parsley
Vermicelli
Seasoning

Cut chicken up into small strips, wash and cover with a little milk for about 15 mins. Wash off the milk.

Place all cleaned and chopped vegetables, bay leaves and chicken in a pot with 3 pints of water.

Cook slowly until everything is tender. You might have to top up the water.

Season to taste with salt and pepper. Remove onion and bay leaves.

The soup can be liquidised or left chunky.

In a separate pot, boil 3 litres of water and when boiling, drop 3 rings of vermicelli pasta. When cooked, strain from water, rinse with cold water and serve with the soup.

QUICK SPINACH SOUP

Donated by Nigella Lawson

Onion, chopped
Spinach, chopped
500ml (1 pint) stock

Lemon juice
Optional – single cream, 1 egg

Spinach, since you can buy it frozen and ready chopped, makes a good basis for a quick soup.

Chop and fry an onion first, then add spinach and when it has more or less thawed, add 500ml or so of stock made from cubes or granules.

After about 5 minutes, add a good squeeze of lemon and if you want to make it thicker when it's off the heat, whisk in some single cream, beaten with an egg yolk.

KAREN'S CHUNKY HADDOCK AND PRAWN SOUP

Donated by Karen Pyke

1 bunch spring onions, trimmed and chopped
1 large potato, peeled and cut into chunks
2 vegetable stock cubes dissolved in 600ml (1 pint) water
350g (12oz) smoked haddock or cod fillet, skinned and cut into chunks

450ml (¾pint) milk
50g (2oz) peas
50g (2oz) peeled prawns
2 tablespoons parsley, chopped
2 level tablespoons cornflour
Salt and freshly ground black pepper

Melt the butter in a large saucepan. Add the spring onions and potato, and cook gently without browning for 5 minutes. Add the stock, bring up to the boil, then reduce the heat. Cover and simmer for about 10 minutes, until the potatoes are almost tender.

Add the fish, milk and peas. Heat and simmer gently until the fish is cooked – about 4 minutes. Next, add the prawns and half the parsley.

Blend the cornflour with 2-3 tablespoons of cold water. Add to the soup and cook gently, stirring all the time, until thickened. Cook gently for another minute or two, then taste and season.

Serve the soup in warmed bowls, garnished with remaining parsley.

Karen also adds:

1 carrot peeled and diced
1 salmon steak, skin removed and diced into 1in pieces

Double quantity of milk and equal amount of single cream
Cream is added after the cornflour

SNAFFLES MOUSSE

300 g (10 oz) Philadelphia cream cheese	1 x 375 g (15 oz) tin Cross and Blackwell consommé
1 x 150 g (6 oz tin) Cambell's consommé – DO NOT CHILL	Garlic salt, pepper and curry paste

Chill the Cross and Blackwell consommé and the cheese. DO NOT CHILL CAMBELL'S CONSOMME.

Put the cheese, ½ of the Cross and Blackwell consommé and all the Cambell's consommé in vegetable mill until smooth.

Add ¼ tsp of curry paste, garlic salt and pepper to taste.

Pour into ramekins and chill for 4 hours.

Decorate with remainder of chilled and chopped consommé or mock caviar or parsley.

AVOCADO SURPRISE

Donated by Jane Garrard
Serves 4

2 avocados	Juice of 1 lemon
135 g (5 oz) cream cheese	Salt and ground pepper
50 g (2 oz) white Chesire or white Stilton cheese, grated	

Remove avocado flesh. Rub skins with lemon juice.

Mix avocado flesh with cream cheese and season to taste.

Place mixture back in skins and sprinkle with grated cheese.

Place under a medium to high grill and cook until cheese has melted.

Serve with walnut bread or rolls as a starter or main course.

TIP! Best with hard skins on the avocados.

HEULYN'S TABOULEH SALAD

This salad should be made with cracked wheat (burghul), but couscous can be used instead. Tomatoes can be added. They make the salad a little mushier.

150 g couscous
1 medium sized onion finely chopped
3 tbsp parsley finely chopped

3 tbsp mint finely chopped
3 tbsp olive oil
Juice of 1 or more lemons, to taste
Salt and pepper

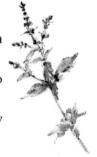

Empty the couscous onto a serving dish.
Cover with ¾ pint of boiling water into which you have mixed a teaspoon of salt.
After a few minutes, fluff up with a fork so that each grain is loose.
Mix with the remaining ingredients and allow to stand for an hour or two before serving.

HEULYN'S EGG MOUSSE

6 eggs
1 tbsp cream or crème fraiche
3-4 tbsp mayonnaise
1 small packet gelatine

2 small tins or 1 jar anchovies
1 tbsp chives
½ cucumber for garnish
Seasoning to taste

Hard boil the eggs, cool, peel and chop.
Mix together cream and mayonnaise.
Crush anchovies and chop chives, (reserving ½ the chives for garnish).
Dissolve gelatine in a little hot water.
Stir all ingredients together and put in lightly oiled ring/mould. Refrigerate until set.

When turning out just before serving, decorate centre with diced cucumber and remaining chives.

TIP! The anchovies are quite salty so seasoning with salt is not recommended.

JUDY'S RECIPE:
BROCCOLI & APPLE PUREE
A WONDERFULLY NUTRITIOUS DISH

2 broccoli heads trimmed and cut into small florets
1 dessert apple quartered and cored
½ lemon
1 tbsp olive oil
2 shallots (or 1 onion) coarsely chopped

150 ml (¼ pint) apple juice
300 ml (½ pint) chicken stock
1tbsp double cream
¼ tsp cinnamon
Salt and freshly ground pepper

Steam the broccoli florets until very soft (about 15 minutes.) Set the broccoli aside.

Reserve 4 thin slices of apple from an apple quarter for garnish and squeeze lemon juice over them to prevent from discolouring.

Peel remaining apple pieces and cut into thin slices.

Put oil in a heavy frying pan over medium heat, add the shallots and cook until they start to look transparent, stir in peeled apple slices, apple juice, stock and bring the liquid to the boil.

Reduce heat and stir until apples are soft, stir in broccoli (reserving 2 florets for garnish) and heat through.

Put the broccoli/apple mixture into a food processor, add cream, cinnamon, salt and pepper, and puree until smooth.

Serve the puree immediately with the reserved broccoli florets and apple slices.

CREAMY WHITE SAUCE

This recipe makes 300 ml (½ pint) and has a million uses in the kitchen.

50 g (2 oz) butter	Salt and freshly ground pepper
1 skinned, finely chopped clove garlic	1 rounded tbsp flour
	300 ml (½ pint) milk
Freshly grated nutmeg	
1 rounded tbsp finely chopped Parsley (optional)	

Melt the butter in a saucepan.
Add finely chopped garlic and flour.
Cook for 2 – 3 minutes, stirring continuously.
Gradually add the milk, beating it in as you go.
Let the sauce boil for a minute, still stirring.
Remove from heat.
Season to taste with salt, pepper, nutmeg and just before serving, stir in the finely chopped parsley.

CAROL'S COMMENT: Parsley is optional – omit it if it creates irritation at the back of the throat.

ONION GRAVY

2 tbsp dripping or 3 tbsp sunflower oil (much nicer with dripping!)	1 rounded tbsp plain flour
	600 ml (1 pint) chicken or vegetable stock
3 onions – skinned and thinly sliced	A few drops of gravy browning if liked

Melt the dripping and onions (if using oil, heat in saucepan before adding onions).

Sauté for 5 – 7 minutes until soft and transparent.

Stir in the flour and cook gently for about 2 more minutes.

Gradually add stock, stirring all the time until gravy boils.

Stir in gravy browning if you are using it.

CAROL'S COMMENT: Delicious with toad-in-the-hole!

SAVOURY LEMON SAUCE

1 onion peeled and finely chopped	4 tbsp dry white wine
Juice of ½ lemon	1 tbsp finely chopped parsley
50 ml (2 oz) chicken stock	50 g (2 oz) butter cut into pieces

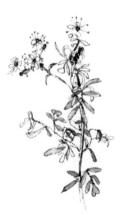

Put the onion into a saucepan, together with the wine and chicken stock.

Bring to a gentle simmering point and continue simmering in an uncovered saucepan until the liquid has reduced by half and the onion is soft.

Whisk in the butter a piece at a time and finally whisk in lemon juice.

Make sure that the liquid does not boil after the butter is added.

Just before serving, whisk in the chopped parsley.

CAROL'S COMMENT: This sauce can be liquidised and is excellent with all grilled fish, meat and chicken, and steamed vegetables.

INGA'S LEMON SOLE FLORENTINE

4 large lemon sole fillets
Juice of ½ a lemon
35 g (1 ½ oz) butter
450 ml (¾ pint) milk

500 g (2 1/2lbs) spinach
25 g (1 oz) grated parmesan cheese
35 g (1 ½ oz) plain flour
Salt and black pepper

Sprinkle the lemon sole with lemon juice, salt and pepper. Fold the fillets in half crosswise and set aside.

Melt the butter in a saucepan, add the flour and cook, stirring for 1 minute.

Remove from heat and gradually blend in the milk, bring to the boil, stirring constantly until the sauce thickens.

Add seasoning to taste.

Wash the spinach, place in a saucepan with no added water (there is enough moisture on the leaves.)

Cook for 2 minutes and drain well.

Stir half of the sauce mixture into the spinach and spoon into a shallow ovenproof dish.

Arrange the fillets on top and sprinkle with parmesan.

Add the remainder of the sauce.

Bake in a preheated oven at 200c or 400f or gas 6 for 30 – 40 minutes.

Tip! Serve with freshly steamed vegetables and mashed potato.

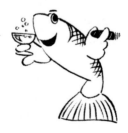

ELSA'S FISH PIE

2 pieces smoked haddock
2 pieces cod
2 pieces fresh salmon
1 packet frozen prawns
1 kg (2.2 lbs) freshly boiled
potatoes
1 bay leaf

1.5 litres (2 pints) milk
100 g (4 oz) butter
100 g (4 oz) plain flour
½ small packet frozen peas
100 g (4 oz) grated cheddar cheese
6 peppercorns

Poach fish for about 5 minutes in milk with bay leaf and peppercorns and leave it to cool in the milk.

Once cool, drain and reserve the milk for the sauce.

Flake the fish, taking care to remove all bones, peppercorns and bay leaf.

Place fish in shallow buttered ovenproof dish.

Add peas and prawns, still frozen.

Melt the butter over a low heat and stir in flour until it thickens.

Gradually stir in the milk until the sauce thickens to a satisfactory consistency (you may have to add more milk if the sauce is too thick).

Add grated cheese to sauce and stir until it melts.

Pour sauce over fish and peas and give it all a gentle stir.

Mash the potatoes with a little milk or cream and spread over the fish.

Dot with butter and place in fairly hot oven for about 20 minutes or until brown on top.

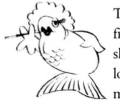

TIP! There is no need to add salt as the smoked fish and cheese are salty enough already. There should be enough sauce to keep the whole dish loose and moist. If it does not seem enough, make more before adding potatoes.

CAULIFLOWER CHEESE

Donated by Nigella Lawson

1 large head of cauliflower
2 bay leaves
110g (4 oz) butter
2 tsps English mustard
50g (2oz) plain flour

500ml milk
275g (11oz) strong cheddar, grated, plus 50g (2oz) for sprinkling on top

Cut the cauliflower into small florets, put into a saucepan with the bay leaves and cover with cold water.

Add a sprinkling of salt and bring to the boil, then drain and refresh with cold water. Let the cauliflower drain again in a colander. Pluck out the bay leaves and discard.

When the cauliflower is completely drained, put into an ovenproof dish in an even layer.

Preheat oven to gas mark 7/220°C.

To make the cheese sauce, melt the butter in a heavily bottomed saucepan, then whisk in the mustard and flour, and cook over a gently heat for about 5 minutes. Whisk in the milk off the heat, then put it back on the heat and keep stirring until it becomes really thick and begins to bubble.

Sprinkle in the 275g grated cheese and stir over the heat until it has melted into the sauce. Check the seasoning, then pour it over the cauliflower in the dish and scatter the remaining cheese over the top.

Cook for 20 minutes at the temperature above, until the cauliflower is hot, the sauce is bubbling and the cheese top is slightly browned.

CAROL'S CREATIONS
LAMB AND ROSEMARY STEW

1.4 kg (3 lbs) lamb neck fillet (or stewing lamb) cut into 5 cm cubes
200 g new potatoes – halved (I sometimes add a sweet potato instead or as well)
300 ml (½ pint) hot lamb or vegetable stock
2 tbsp olive oil

2 tbsp plain flour
4 tbsp freshly chopped rosemary
1 small swede – chopped
1 tbsp tomato puree
2 sliced red onions
1 small aubergine – chopped
Large handful spinach (optional)

Heat the oil in a large pan over a medium heat.
Put the lamb in a bowl, add the flour and rosemary, season and toss to coat the meat.
Fry the lamb in batches for 5 minutes until browned all over. Remove from the pan and set aside.
Add the onions, swede, aubergine and potatoes to the pan. Fry for 10 minutes until golden brown.
Return the lamb to the pan with the tomato puree and stock. Cover, bring to the boil and simmer for about 1 hour until the lamb is tender.
Remove lid and cook for a further 15 minutes to thicken the sauce.

Alternatively – put the lamb into a casserole dish and cover with foil.
Put into a preheated oven (150C) and cook slowly for 1 ½ to 2 ½ hours.
Remove foil 15 minutes before end of cooking time.

Add spinach and allow to wilt.

TIP! Serve with a dollop of natural yoghurt or cream or soured cream if desired. Freezes well.

PUDDINGS:

LEMON MERINGUE ICE-CREAM

Donated by Nigella Lawson

600ml whipping cream   2 lemons, juice and zest
225g (9oz) Greek yoghurt   6 meringue nests
320g (12-13oz) lemon curd

Whip the cream until fairly stiff and fold in the yoghurt.
Add the lemon curd, lemon juice and zest (you will find it easier to stir in the curd if you add the lemon juice first) and the meringues, broken into small pieces, but not so small that they'll dissolve into dust.
Put into a container – it should be a shallow rather than a tall one. Freeze the mixture and that's all there is to it.
Ripen in the fridge for 40 minutes before you want to eat it.
If preferred, dribble some clear honey or some more lemon curd diluted to runniness with the lemon juice.

Another idea:
Make a pavlova base and smear with some thickly whipped cream. Then thickly cover that with lemon curd and even more thickly with more whipped cream, and dot with raspberries.

ICED ORANGE AND APRICOT MOUSSE

Dinner/lunch party – serves 8

250 g (10 oz) apricots
Pared rind of 1 orange
50 g (2 oz) sieved icing sugar
Juice of 2 oranges

3 eggs – separated
300 ml (½ pint) double cream
3 – 4 tbsp orange liqueur

Put the apricots in a saucepan, together with the orange juice and rind.

(Use potato peeler to pare the rind as thinly as possible.)

Simmer gently until the apricots are soft. Run apricots through a sieve to get a smooth puree. Leave to cool.

Whisk the egg yolks until stiff. Gradually whisk in sieved icing sugar – a spoonful at a time until you have a stiff meringue.

Whip the cream and orange liqueur together.

Fold the apricot puree into the whipped cream.

Fold the stiff egg yolk mixture into the apricot cream.

Using a metal spoon, fold the meringue mixture into the apricot mixture and place the whole thing into a large plastic container.

Seal and freeze.

Remove from freezer 20 – 25 minutes before serving and keep at room temperature.

Scoop out into a chilled bowl to serve.

VANILLA CUSTARD

Makes 600 ml (1 pint)

600 ml (1 pint) milk
4 large egg yolks
1 tsp sieved cornflour

50 g (2 oz) sugar
½ tsp vanilla essence

Put milk in a saucepan over a moderate heat.
Beat together the egg yolk, cornflour and caster sugar.
Beat a little of the hot milk into the yolk mixture and return to the milk in the saucepan.
Stir over a gentle heat until the sauce coats the back of a wooden spoon, sufficiently thick enough for you to draw a line down the middle of the spoon with your finger.
Remove from heat and stir in vanilla essence.
Serve warm.

CAROL'S COMMENTS: This custard goes well with any steamed pudding and is the vital ingredient in any 'proper' trifle.

JANE'S APPLE BRULEE

500 g (1 lb) cooking apples
50 g (2 oz) sugar
50 g (2 oz) brown sugar

Large tub natural yoghurt or mixture of cream, yoghurt or crème fraiche

Peel apples and cook down to a pulp. Sweeten to taste and place in shallow dish.
Cover with yoghurt or cream mixture.
Sprinkle with brown sugar and leave in fridge overnight.

APRICOT CRUMBLE

1 tin apricots in natural juice
200 g (8 oz) plain flour
100 g (4 oz) muesli (optional)

75 g (3 oz) sugar – caster or granulated

Put apricots in bottom of an ovenproof dish with some of the juice.

171

Make the crumble by mixing the flour and butter together in a bowl until you have a consistency resembling fine breadcrumbs.

Add sugar to the mixture, as well as muesli if desired.

Pour the crumble mix over the apricots and place in a preheated oven (180C) for about 45 minutes.

Tip! Delicious with custard and/or ice cream.

VANESSA'S BLUEBERRY AND LAVENDER JELLY

This delicious recipe has blueberries which are full of antioxidants and the cheese provides calcium, while the lavender lifts the spirits.

4/5 stems fresh lavender or 1 teaspoon of dried lavender
600 ml (1 pint) blueberry juice

Mascarpone cheese
Gelatine

Infuse the lavender and blueberry juice, warming gently – be careful not to boil.

Leave for between 30 minutes and 8 hours depending on how strong you like the lavender to be. Strain.

Warm the blueberry and lavender infusion and add gelatine, following manufacturer's instructions.

Pour into 4 pretty glasses and chill in fridge until set.

When set, put a large dollop of mascarpone cheese on top and decorate with fresh lavender.

Serve chilled.

ELSA'S SLURPY PUDDING

Sliced soft summer fruits (e.g. mango and oranges) or cold stewed fruit (e.g. rhubarb or apple)

Large carton of yoghurt or crème fraiche
Soft dark brown sugar

Place the fruit on a flattish dish or flan and cover it with the yoghurt or crème fraiche.

Sprinkle a generous amount of brown sugar over the top and set aside in the fridge, preferably overnight, to allow the sugar to sink down and flavour the whole dish.

DAVID'S DELIGHT! GINGERBREAD

Enough for one 900 g (2 lb) loaf

100 g (4 oz)soft light brown sugar
75 g (3 oz) golden syrup
105 ml (7 tbsp) semi-skimmed milk
150 g (6 oz) gluten-free plain flour
Pinch of salt
7.5 ml (1 ½ tsp) gluten-free baking powder

75 g (3oz) soft margarine
75 g (3 oz) black treacle
1 beaten egg
50 g (2 oz) gram flour
10 ml (2 tsp) ground ginger
5 ml (1 tsp) ground cinnamon

Preheat the oven to 160c/325f/gas 3.

Lightly grease and line a 900 g (2 lb) loaf tin.

Place the sugar, margarine, syrup and treacle in a saucepan and heat gently until melted and blended, stirring occasionally. Remove the pan from the heat, leave to cool slightly, then mix in the milk and egg.

Mix the flours, salt, spices and baking powder in a large bowl.

Make a well in the centre, pour in the liquid mixture and beat well.

Pour the contents of the mixture into the prepared loaf tin and bake for 1 – 1 ¼ hours until firm to the touch and lightly browned.

Allow to cool in the tin for a few minutes, then turn out onto a rack to cool completely.

Store in an airtight container.

Chapter 7

THE DUNSTONE BENNETT COMPLEMENTARY CENTRE

The DB centre is open three days a week: Tuesday, 9.30am to 2.30pm; Wednesday, 9.30am to 12.30pm and Thursday between 9.30am and 2.30pm.

For enquiries or to book an appointment, please ring 07541 998711 or 01604 635889 or visit the website www.facefax.org.uk

The Dunstone Bennett Complementary Centre,
The Basement Suite,
38 Billing Road,
Northampton
NN1 5DQ

Anne Hicks RGN, BSc(Hons)
Maxillofacial Clinical Nurse Specialist & Chairperson of Facefax

I have worked in Head & Neck Oncology for fifteen years, both in theatres as a scrub nurse and in Outpatient Clinics. I meet people from all walks of life, aged from mid-twenties to very elderly. I am with my patients and their families/friends/carers from the point of diagnosis to five years post treatment, at which time they are statistically cured of the treated cancer.

I am in a very privileged position whereby I see patients in a clinical setting at Northampton General Hospital (NGH), as well as in my role of Chairperson of Facefax. I actively support and encourage the wonderful work taking place in the Dunstone Bennett Complementary Therapy Centre (DB), which also welcomes carers and family members.

I have no doubt that everyone who attends for a treatment benefits. Patients can often feel deserted by the clinical team once their treatment is finished, leaving them to manage a variety of symptoms alone. There is always support available at the end of a phone, but the patients have to actually pick up the phone! The conversation usually starts with "I am sorry to bother you, I know how busy you are..." They worry that their concerns are trivial compared to having major surgery or chemo-radiotherapy.

However, it is at this point when the DB Centre becomes invaluable. The volunteers have been with us for several years and are extremely good at managing some very difficult conversations with distressed patients or carers. The DB Centre has a feeling of calm that has to be experienced to be understood, and this is created by those volunteers running it.

People benefit in a variety of ways; they are able to talk freely about their treatment without worrying about what their significant others will think. They are able to relax during Reiki or Massage sessions and often say they feel better for days afterwards. They report a reduction in pain and discomfort and this helps them to get a good night's sleep. This helps to maintain a positive attitude, which can sometimes be difficult when struggling to cope with a life-changing experience. Those people who are able to remain positive and upbeat will still have their dark moments, but these will be short-lived, and other people will be more likely to want to be around them, which helps them to keep busy and occupy their minds.

Everyone will cope in a different way, but those people who

choose to attend the DB Centre tend to keep coming back as it is beneficial to them – this particularly includes carers, who can get overlooked by the clinical team. Watching someone you love go through major surgery or other cancer treatments can be emotionally draining and sometimes heartbreaking, so these people need support too. I attend myself as often as I can because... nurses are only human and we get exhausted, too!

Christine Gould,
Centre Manager & Therapist

Bridging the gap between science and spirituality was the mission of Carol Dunstone and Ann Bennett following their recovery from cancer – and four years ago, they created The DB. The continuing success of the centre depends on good practice, the close working partnership with medical staff at Northampton General Hospital, support from Macmillan, donations, and a wonderful team of volunteers.

The aim of the centre is to help and support patients, carers, relatives and friends at any stage of their journey through cancer by offering a choice of therapies, advice and education. It is clear that for many people it has become a sanctuary at a time of personal difficulty. Complementary therapies are natural, holistic treatments that are regularly used in addition to conventional medical practices.

This integrated approach to healthcare is not new and one which both Ann Bennett and I have been involved with for many years. It follows on from the work carried out at the Pain Relief Clinic, NGH, in the 1990s, when, alongside conventional medicine, consultants and staff regularly treated patients with acupuncture, massage and other complementary strategies.

Giving talks to groups attending the Pain Management Course and carrying out Reiki treatments and Spiritual Healing was part of Ann's contribution. Christine was a member of the multidisciplinary team, supporting those suffering with chronic pain by the application of self-hypnosis and relaxation.

The centre has a network of volunteers and, supported by Ann and Christine, they bring to the centre a variety of skills including Reiki, reflexology and Indian head massage; neck, shoulder and back massage; counselling; beauty treatment and advice; art therapy and legal advice. Three volunteers are responsible for the day-to-day running of the centre and they organise the rota for the other volunteer therapists and receptionists.

Building on the professional relationships established with NGH staff, paved the way for the organisation to work within the hospital supporting oncology patients and their families, particularly those attending the Children's Outpatients Department. The Disney Team, as it is now called, has seven volunteer therapists from the centre who have previous experience working in a medical environment – others, with children.

It may take weeks, even months, for a potential client to pluck up the courage to make that initial phone call to the centre and we are aware that every effort must be made to minimise this anxiety. With this in mind, all calls are answered during working hours, thereby eliminating the need to leave a message. This is particularly important for those who have had recent surgery and may find speech difficult.

Initially, a client is asked to visit the centre, meet one of the team and complete a questionnaire, so that we are fully aware of their needs and most importantly the therapies which may assist their recovery. After this, an optional hands on healing treatment of Reiki is offered. Clients are also welcome to bring along a loved one or friend who can also receive a therapy of their choice – subject only to their medical condition.

The number of visits to the centre by cancer patients, relatives and carers, varies according to need. Some clients attend weekly; others, every fortnight or month. All receive the same high standard of treatment and feedback is requested so we can monitor and improve our performance. After treatment, many of our clients report increased energy levels, an improved quality of life, and reduced feelings of isolation. Others develop a more positive attitude to recover from their condition.

Following a successful laryngectomy, Mick, aged sixty-eight, was encouraged by a regular client to come along and experience a Reiki treatment. Unsure what to expect, he was surprised how relaxing and calming the effects were. Feeling so much better, he has continued to attend every week for almost two years. He has now become an advocate for the centre and also visits patients during their stay at NGH.

His wife, Jean, noticed the gradual changes and, intrigued by his progress, decided to book a Reiki treatment. This also gave her the opportunity to meet the therapists Mick fondly talked about. Jean described feeling "wonderful, extremely relaxed and relieved of stress from a busy time at work."

Attractive young mum, Mandy, aged forty, turned to complementary therapy when diagnosed with breast cancer and wasn't thrilled at the prospect of losing her hair. Impressed by our support, half the proceeds from a ball she is organising are destined for The DB. Mandy went on to say, "It helped keep me sane when

I was at the darkest days of my life. I will always be thankful for how much you've helped me. I am now back at work and still have a full head of hair."

Evelyn, aged fifty-six, whose health has improved considerably since visiting the centre, said "It's a fantastic place and takes me out of myself. Everyone is so friendly; they really listen to me and are genuinely interested in my progress."

For Janet, aged fifty-two, the centre has provided a place for her teenage son, Adam, to get the help and support needed after his father's passing. Adam was able to talk to someone who could understand what he was going through, take notice of him and how he was feeling. Whereas for Janet, it gave her somewhere to look forward to going each week and helped her deal with the grief of being separated from her husband.

Carol Dunstone
Art Therapist & Facefax Trustee

As a ceramic artist and painter, I thought it would be a wonderful idea if we could set up an Art Therapy Day at the DB, for the benefit of cancer patients, carers and relatives.

Creativity is such a stress buster – so much so, that I really do believe anyone, whether they can paint or not, can always find a way to express themselves. The Art Day was set up in 2009 and has proved to be hugely popular and successful. Everyone who attends arrives with enthusiasm, but not necessarily any experience. This does not matter, as most importantly it is a gathering for sharing experiences, which is a therapy in itself.

All this would be impossible without Jean, a valued member of the management team, who provides help and encouragement, especially with lending a supportive ear to anyone who might be having a 'down' day. Her help is invaluable. The Art Class is very positive and we do have quite a lively time, with much discussion and laughter. All those who come find it very refreshing and they forget for a while about other matters that might be concerning them.

We have lots of different projects on the go, such as ceramic painting, watercolour painting, modelling in clay, discussions on photography, stencilling and many other ideas. Most of the art materials are provided for the class, which is a great help.

Another dear friend of mine, Elke Pollard, who is an accomplished artist in her own right, comes along to help – adding another dimension to the class. Also, not forgetting my sculptor husband, who has happily stepped in to support us all as well.

The Art Therapy Day is a very happy day and has certainly proved to be very positive for all those who attend during the various stages of their cancer journey. It is run entirely on a voluntary basis, while a small donation towards the running costs of the DB Centre is always welcome.

My personal work as a volunteer at the DB Centre has given me an incredible sense of fulfilment, which has sustained my belief in the purpose of all the energetic and devoted work that is being achieved at the centre for cancer patients.

Jean Patchesa
Facefax Trustee & Therapist

I was introduced to the Facefax members by Anne Hicks, soon after my husband, sadly, lost his life to mouth cancer. At the time I felt I needed to meet some people who had gone through the same treatments as he had and to meet those who survived, as I felt it may help my grieving process.

When I joined, Ann and Carol had written their first book and were just talking about their new project – a Complementary Therapy Centre for patients, their carers and families (an idea I applauded) who were being treated in NGH for any type of cancer. I wanted to help, although I was a little unsure if my story would make it hard for them to find a place for me.

Gladly, I was welcomed with open arms and have been with them ever since. I started working weekly with Ann as a receptionist, helped Carol with her Art Day once a month and I was invited to become a Trustee after a while.

Having never heard of Reiki, our clients' amazing transformations after just one treatment persuaded me to try it myself. After just half an hour, I was hooked. I took my Reiki 1 and soon after Reiki 11, then I got myself insured and am now able to offer myself as a therapist, along with being a member of the management team and a receptionist. Oh yes, and I do laundry, banking and stock control too – not "Jack" but "Jean of all Trades".

My introduction to Facefax and Dunstone Bennett was so sad, but I feel really privileged to have met and worked with such a wonderful group of people. The therapists, receptionists and clients are all very special to me and I have loved the time I have spent to date with them all. Long may it continue.

Joyce Turner
Carer, Facefax Secretary & Trustee

My partner Doug was diagnosed with mouth and neck cancer in September 2007. Doug had major surgery, chemotherapy and radiotherapy over a period of six months and then had further surgery over the next few years. The good news was that Mr Harrop, Max Fax Consultant, saved Doug's tongue.

All this was happening whilst I was holding down a very demanding consultancy job with very tight timescales. My career had spanned forty-two years – time to give it up and have a major rethink. My job would be disappearing within a year, so I negotiated a redundancy package two years before I officially retired at sixty. Now, what to do with my time in-between caring for Doug and driving to a variety of hospitals etc.?

A letter dropped on the mat just as I started my redundancy. It was from Anne Hicks, a Specialist Clinical Nurse at the maxillofacial unit, inviting Doug and me to join the Facefax Charity and meet people who had gone through similar experiences. I thought "Why not?" I probably had something to offer, but more importantly, I could meet other people who had experienced a cancer journey. Sometimes, as a carer, it can be quite scary and lonely, not knowing if you are doing the right thing. Doug did not want to join; he did not want to relive his experiences, he just wanted to move on. I fully understood and accepted that; however, Doug understood why it might help me.

As a carer, through the whole journey and now, I thought I might lose Doug. We also had questions like would he still be able to talk after the operation? Doug is extremely quick-witted and funny, but would he lose this? Would his personality change? What would he be able to eat? As chef of the house, how would

Doug cope if he could not taste? Would he be able to work again? How would I be able to cope without him? How would I be able to cope with the unknown, as I am not a 'natural' carer but, a more practical doer?

I needed support and found the charity a gift and a blessing. The meetings were also social. These volunteers had experienced what I had and had moved on, were enjoying life and managing day-to-day challenges with a positive outlook. I was able to share their experiences and suggestions with Doug, which helped with managing lack of saliva, swallowing and pains in the arms etc.

We now have a strong circle of supportive friends and I have since become the Facefax Secretary and Trustee. It has been an amazing journey, which is still ongoing, and I hope I have been able to help others along the way as much as Doug and I have been helped.

Thank you.

ALDERWOOD
LIVING AND LEARNING WITH AUTISM MEETS FACEFAX

G Birse, Alderwood LLA

I am not sure if it was fate or pure coincidence that myself and a colleague from Alderwood LLA were introduced to Facefax. The first time we had heard of Facefax was during a social gathering, which Ann Bennett also attended. It was during a conversation that Ann started to tell my colleague and I about the Dunstone and Bennett Complementary Therapy Centre, and how Ann and Carol, the founders of this remarkable service, had links from their personal experiences with cancer. I think once you hear how these wonderful ladies conquered their own battles with cancer and then went on to initiate and create the Complementary Therapy Centre, you can't help but want to get involved in some way – no matter how small or large it may seem.

Anita Smart (Strategic Director at Alderwood LLA) immediately felt Alderwood LLA could in some way, through their charitable board, support the centre and introduced Facefax to the Alderwood LLA fundraising group. Fundraising was soon put into operation and included selling quiz sheets, magazines, book and DVD sales, raffles, tea and coffee sales, and monthly employee donations direct from their wages. The money raised allowed us to support the DB almost straightaway. That was two years ago and we are still passionate about supporting the centre as much as we can. Visitors to the centre and fundraising events held by Facefax cemented the importance of the service this centre continually provides for patients and families touched by facial and head cancer. During the last year or so, I have been fortunate to meet the volunteer therapists and the hub of operations, Ann, Carol, Joyce and the wonderful receptionists, who ensure this charity is run with the patients' needs being paramount; a truly humbling team of amazing ladies.

It wasn't long before staff members at Alderwood were asking about our chosen charity for 2011/2012 and a number of them donated funds raised from their own car boot sales etc. In 2012, changes for the centre seemed to be heading towards the therapists extending their services to the Disney Ward of Northampton General Hospital. Alderwood LLA was able to assist by covering the costs involved for the DBS checks that were required for the ever growing number of therapists. Our relationship has grown and it is always good to drop in and catch up with a few of the ladies from the DB.

Alderwood have continued to pass on the awareness of head and facial cancer and how the DB support their patients. It is important to Alderwood that we introduce all new employees to the charities we have been involved with over the last ten years and by doing so, they have access to our charity display boards where Facefax is currently exhibited. The information gives staff an insight into the work carried out and the availability of this service – which is on our very own doorstep. As fate would have it and unknown to us at the time in 2011, some of us have close family members and friends who have since experienced cancer themselves. This makes fundraising for Facefax even more poignant.

The awareness of facial and head cancer would be lessoned without this wonderful organisation. With virtually non-existent government funding, it is left to this dedicated team and their charity fundraisers to meet the annual running costs for the centre and to continue its journey forward. It has always been apparent that during this constant struggle for funding, the DB's number one priority is to meet the needs of the people touched emotionally or physically by cancer. There are seldom times in our lives when we can say we have met people who are truly inspirational. Alderwood were introduced to a whole group of these people back in 2011 and we feel privileged to have been given the chance to get to know them personally, while gaining an insight into the wonderful service they provide.

Lisa Mullins
Macmillan Regional Involvement Coordinator

I am grateful to have this opportunity to thank Ann and Carol for their commitment and dedication, both in supporting Macmillan and in making a difference to the lives of people affected by cancer.

It's a testament to the character of both these women that they took something as tough as a cancer diagnosis and used their experiences to make a positive difference to other people's lives.

Setting up the Dunstone Bennett Complementary Therapy Centre and a Head and Neck Support Group in Northamptonshire has given cancer patients and their families a safe haven to get away from the physical and emotional stress that comes with a cancer diagnosis. The centre has gone from strength to strength, thanks to the enthusiasm, dedication and devotion of both women and loyal, committed volunteers.

They have also played a vital role in improving cancer care and services for local people by working with Macmillan to look at how we can develop, improve and redesign services over the next three years for patients with head and neck cancers, to ensure they get the best possible quality of care and support. The treatment of these cancers can often involve complex surgery and radiotherapy, which can have significant physical and psychosocial effects on patients and their families.

No one should face cancer alone and with the support of dynamic and inspirational people like Ann and Carol, no one will have to.

Jane Tebbutt
Children's Outreach Macmillan Nurse

Children's cancers are rare compared to adult cancers, with an estimated incidence of one in every 500 children aged under fifteen years being diagnosed with cancer each year. [Macmillan 2012].

This means that approximately 1700 children in the UK and between fifteen to twenty children locally [Northamptonshire] will have a new cancer diagnosis each year.

Children's cancers are usually different in type from the cancers affecting adults and because of this, they react differently to treatments.

It is expected that approximately 75% of all children with cancer will be cured and for some types of childhood cancers, such as Acute Lymphoblastic Leukaemia, the expected cure rate is much higher.

As the numbers of children with cancer are small compared to the adult population with cancer, hospital care is organised and provided differently.

Care in the UK is organised and supervised by one of the twenty-one Children's Cancer and Leukaemia Group Centres. These centres operate as 'Principle Treatment Centres [PTCs] to co-ordinate and supervise patient treatments, and advise on training and accreditation.

Currently, the PTC used by children and families in Northamptonshire is the Queens Medical Centre in Nottingham.

The PCTs then work with other hospitals, such as Northampton General Hospital, on a 'shared care' basis to provide 'care nearer to home'.

The level of 'shared care' a hospital can provide is assessed annually according to recommendations arising from the document *Improving Outcomes Guidance for Children and Young People with Cancer* [NICE 2005].

Northampton General Hospital's, Disney Ward has been assessed to provide the highest level of care [Level 3] which can be given outside the PTC.

A specially trained team of doctors, nurses, play specialists and teachers are based on Disney Ward to provide care to children with cancer and their families, in a range of settings [hospital, outpatients and home], to provide a flexible and holistic service for all.

Cancer Geneticist
Dr. Julian Barwell
University Hospitals of Leceister NHS Trust

I was delighted to have the opportunity to say a few words in this book about familial cancer susceptibility and partnerships in healthcare.

Cancer is becoming an increasing problem worldwide and this is largely through the westernisation of cultures, resulting in smoking and alcohol consumption, dietary choices that lead to obesity. Changes to the genetic code occur in all tumours, but the vast majority of these are not inherited. Approximately 1% of individuals have inherited an alteration in a gene (an instruction to help build and repair our bodies), which greatly increases their risk of cancer. At the clinical genetics department at the Leicester Royal Infirmary we have tried to simplify our advice using a 3,2,1 rule: if three members of the family are affected, across two generations and one was diagnosed under the age of fifty, it is worth asking your doctor if there could be a link.

Latest evidence also suggests that even individuals without a family history of cancer, but have been diagnosed with a hormonal unresponsive breast cancer or bowel cancer under the age of fifty, may have an inherited alteration in a cancer susceptibility gene. This is becoming increasingly important as the opportunities for screening are improving. There is growing evidence that active lifestyle choices, preventative surgery and chemoprevention can reduce the risk of cancer. Genetics is rapidly improving our understanding of a number of these diseases.

There is no doubt in my mind that modern medicine does not have all the answers and we all need to work more closely to support and protect families affected by cancer. We do this in

Leicester by running outreach events in the community and inviting dieticians, physiotherapists, specialist nurses, surgeons, psychotherapists, researchers and research networks, local and national patient support groups and patients.

I hope you enjoy the book and it helps families on their cancer journey.

Chapter 8

CONTACTS AND REFERRALS

This chapter lists the contact numbers, addresses and websites for therapists, medical specialists and products mentioned in this book, along with other useful numbers and websites connected with these particular areas.

Please note that clients are advised to seek medical attention before making an appointment to see a complementary therapist.

Arnica Gel:
For information on this massage gel, visit www.qvcuk.com. The order line is 0800 504030

Coconut Oil:
Details of this nutritious oil can be found at Coconut Connections, www.coconut-connections.com

COMPLEMENTARY THERAPIES:

Aromatherapy and Reflexology
Tel: 01604 757771
Website: www.studio-53.co.uk

Hypnotherapy
Tel: 01604 624515

Email: info@christinegould.com
Websites: www.christinegould.com
www.atkinsonballcollege.com

Reiki
To learn more about the original Usui Shiki Ryoho tradition of Reiki in its purest form, contact Rei-ki Academy: 01604 624515
Email: reikiacademycg@gmail.com
Website: www.christinegould.com

To find a qualified healer in your area, contact:

> The Holistic Energy Association,
> The Lodge,
> Mount Pleasant Road,
> Lindford,
> Hampshire GU35 0PR

Email: contact@holisticenergyassociation.com
Website: www.theholisticenergyassociation.com

Cymatherapy
For further information about Energetic Bioresonance Rebalancing, consult Cymatherapy Practitioner Christine Gould
Tel: 01604 624515
Email: info@christinegould.com
Website: www.christinegould.com

Transference Healing
For more information, contact Sandy Reygan
Tel: 07861 943261

Email: genna2win@yahoo.co.uk
Website: www.sandyreygan.com

Hair and Beauty
Michele Dupuy-Sherratt. Midus Health and Beauty.
Tel: 07939580023

The Hair and Beauty Service
You can contact Deborah Smith, from the Hair and Beauty Service, on Tel: 01604 544486

Counselling Therapy:
Yvonne Miller, Dip Cou Studies, Dip NLP E.M.D.R Therapy.
Tel (07940)544042

Diet:
World Cancer Research has a good deal of information on diet and health guidelines for cancer prevention: www.wcrf-k.org

Dry Mouth Care Products:
Biotene Dry Mouth Care Mouthwash.
Biotene Oral Balance Saliva Replacement Gel.
Biotene Oral Dry Mouth Toothpaste.
Biotene Anti-Bacterial Dry Mouth Gum.
Xerotin
Duraphat Fluoride Toothpaste
GC Tooth Mousse (Topical cream with bio-available calcium and phosphate).
All the above can be available on prescription.

ONCOLOGY:

Pauline Gibbings.
Macmillan Head and Neck Clinical Nurse Specialist. Head and Neck Unit, ENT, Outpatients Department, Cliftonville, Northampton, NN1 5BD. Direct line: (01604) 523860.

Macmillan Cancer Information & Support Centre,
Northamptonshire Centre for Oncology, Northampton General Hospital, Cliftonville, Northampton, NN1 5BD.
Tel: (01604) 544211

Macmillan Cancer Support
Freephone: 0808 808 0000
Website: www.macmillan.org.uk,
Email: cancerline@macmillan.org.uk

NHS
Website: www.incancernetwork.nhs.uk

Cancer BACUP.
For information, help and support about all aspects of cancer.
Freephone: 0808 800 1234. www.cancerbacup.org.uk
Rarer Cancer Forum. www.rarercancers.org.uk

Oncology Hair Care Advisor.
Hair and Beauty Service. Northampton General Hospital.
Tel: (01604) 544486.

Look Good – Feel Better.
Helping to improve the quality of life for women living with cancer.
At Oxford: Maggies Cancer Information, Churchill Hospital.
Tel: (01865) 225690.

At Cambridge: Addenbrookes Hospital.
Tel: (01223) 216313

Changing Faces, London.
The way you face disfigurement.
Email: info@changingfaces.org.uk
Website: www.changingfaces.org.uk

World Cancer Research (WCRF UK)
    19, Harley Street,
    London,
    WIG 9QJ
Tel: (0207) 3434205
Fax: 0207344201

ORGANIC AND OTHER HEALTH FOODS:

Health Quest(for your healthy lifestyle)
    Grosvenor Centre,
    8 Wood Street,
    Northampton,
    NN1 2ED.
Tel: (01604) 630125 or 07738 556665.

The Facefax Association
Charity for Mouth, Head and Neck Cancer
Website: www.Facefax.org.uk

The Dunstone Bennett Complementary Centre,
    The Basement Suite,
    38 Billing Road, Northampton,
    NN1 5DQ.
Tel: 07541998711 or 01604 635889

CHAPTER 9

THE FACEFAX ASSOCIATION

The Facefax Association aims to raise the profile of maxillofacial units and the treatment of face, head and neck cancers by representing patients and treatments available in Northamptonshire.

Facefax aims to promote the self-awareness and self-examination that leads to early diagnosis, referral and treatment. It will do this by networking information through local support groups attached to all NHS maxillofacial surgical units and any other NHS surgical units treating head and neck cancer.

The association supports patients by promoting their physical and mental health before surgery and during rehabilitation. This can be done through education and practical advice. Patients may be given further aid after maxillofacial surgery, chemotherapy or radiotherapy from facilities, support services and equipment not normally provided by the NHS.

Carers in the family are supported with advice and education on how to apply specialised care techniques.

To support these aims, Facefax produces leaflets and booklets for patients or their advisors to help those who have had maxillofacial surgery, particularly reconstructive surgery. This support is directly available to support groups nationwide, which will in turn, support the patients and carers in their local group.

Where necessary, Facefax will help provide domestic or personal equipment to aid the patient in eating or communicating and in their physical well-being.

The Facefax Association can provide specialist counselling, training and hands-on instruction for carers, supported with suitable documentation. It can provide limited financial aid, if specified by the trustees, to help local support groups operate satisfactorily.

On the professional front, Facefax can enable staff at maxillofacial units to further their education and provide further research into treatment. It will aim to motivate and promote research into prevention, treatment and aftercare, together with the supply of specialised equipment.

This will be achieved by providing funds, when available, for educating and training medical or nursing personnel. This would be in specialised subjects or techniques that help maxillofacial patients and are not normally covered.

For more information, visit our website: www.Facefax.org.uk

POSTSCRIPT

Ann Bennett was determined that she and Carol Dunstone would finish this book, even though she was suffering from a recurrence of cancer.

She worked bravely and tirelessly to complete it, but sadly lost her fight for life on February 28th 2014, just days after signing off the final proofs.